Palgrave Studies in Prisons and Penology

This is a unique and innovative series, the first of its kind dedicated entirely to prison scholarship. At a historical point in which the prison population has reached an all-time high, the series seeks to analyse the form, nature and consequences of incarceration and related forms of punishment. Palgrave Studies in Prisons and Penology provides an important forum for burgeoning prison research across the world.

More information about this series at
http://www.palgrave.com/gp/series/14596

Landon Kuester

Violence in Pursuit of Health

Living with HIV in the American Prison System

palgrave
macmillan

Landon Kuester
King's College London
London, UK

Palgrave Studies in Prisons and Penology
ISBN 978-3-030-61349-5 ISBN 978-3-030-61350-1 (eBook)
https://doi.org/10.1007/978-3-030-61350-1

This Palgrave Macmillan imprint is published by the registered company Springer Nature Switzerland AG
The registered company address is: Gewerbestrasse 11, 6330 Cham, Switzerland

Acknowledgments

This book offers findings from an ethnographic study in a U.S. state prison system. The research involved spending extended time in several prison facilities and community organisations to understand the experiences of people living with HIV as they move through prison and return to life in the community.

Writing this book would not be possible without the generosity and thoughtfulness of all the research participants involved in the study. Therefore, I would like to thank the inmates, prison staff and administrators, ex-inmates and their families, university faculty, hospital staff, social workers, outreach workers, probation and parole board, and leadership at the Department of Health who shared their stories with me.

Research for this book was undertaken as part of my doctoral studies at the London School of Hygiene & Tropical Medicine, University of London. A special thank you is due to Professor Tim Rhodes for his supervision and to advisory committee members Dr. Nicki Thorogood, Professor Ernest Drucker, and Dr. Magdalena Harris. Professor Adam Fletcher guided initial stages of research. The doctoral thesis was examined by Professor Fiona Measham and Dr. Michael Shiner, who provided thoughtful feedback to strengthen this work.

The research would not have been possible without the extraordinary mentorship from Professor Josiah Rich and Professor Tim Flannigan. I would also like to thank Professor Lina Fruzzetti, Dr. Patricia Symonds, and Professor Judith Green. Their support and kindness were immeasurable throughout this study.

I am grateful for the encouragement and support of Dr. Catherine McGowan and Dr. Shirley Huchcroft, interview transcription by Ms. Sally Read, and the generous review and feedback offered by Ms. Sheena Stapleton, Ms. Brieann Buckley, and Ms. Ana Sanandres.

The research underpinning this book was conducted a few years ago now, and several other people have been integral to its production. Professor Kamaldeep Bhui, Professor Simon Dein, and Dr. Mark Freestone encouraged the book submission and guided me through the development of its proposal. I am also grateful to Dr. Polly Radcliffe for her support during the final stages of the write-up.

Some of the analysis in the book reworks previously published material, and therefore I am grateful to the publishers for their permissions to re-produce it here.

Chapter 4 & Discussion: Kuester, L. B., & Freestone, M. C. (2020). Time away is time out: narratives of intentional reimprisonment amongst inmates living with HIV in a US setting. Critical Public Health, 1–12. https://doi.org/10.1080/09581596.2020.1737645.

I dedicate this book to Angel and Big Jay, two participants who died during the course of this study. It was an honour and privilege to have spent time with them both. I will forever hold their stories in my heart and mind, and I hope this book does justice to their experiences.

Contents

List of Tables

1

Introduction: Violence in Pursuit of Health

I felt nervous sitting in the passenger seat of Dr. McGreevy's minivan as he peeled out from the hospital parking lot and raced toward the prison. As we moved through traffic, I tried to wipe the sweat from my hands. The anticipation and anxiety of meeting inmates had become far too real. McGreevy, who seemed unaware of my discomfort, handed me a bible and asked me to recite a morning prayer. I chirped "Awake, my glory, Awake, O-harp and lyre, I will awake the dawn" Dr. McGreevy, an HIV specialist consulting the state prison system, invited me to observe his clinical consultations with inmates. This was my first opportunity to experience life behind bars. On this morning we rushed to meet inmates before officers conducted their morning count, a human inventory that temporarily restricts inmates from coming and going to the medical dispensary.

The heavy door hissed and clanked, rolled back, and I entered the central courtyard of Men's Medium Security Prison. Appearing before me were hundreds of inmates dressed in tan uniforms. While some of the men did pull-ups and lifted weights, others reclined in the grass or walked circles along the perimeter. There was no longer a comfortable distance between myself and the plight of the so-called 'criminal justice-involved population', which, up until this point, I could only sympathise with

L. Kuester, *Violence in Pursuit of Health*, Palgrave Studies in Prisons and Penology, https://doi.org/10.1007/978-3-030-61350-1_1

through media reports and academic texts. Nothing could have prepared me for my first glimpse of mass incarceration. Even now, after spending hundreds of hours inside the prison system, I struggle to comprehend the sheer size of this human experiment.

This book presents research that explored the "lived experience" of 34 male and female inmates living with the human immunodeficiency virus (HIV) as they progressed through a combined U.S. state jail-prison system[1] and into the community. The study of HIV-positive inmates offered a point of entry into understanding how "violence" was situationally created and reproduced between inmates and a range of medical, social welfare, and security staff. Therefore, this book documents the way HIV-positive inmates went about achieving agency through harm to their body and social standing in order to improve their health under conditions of remarkable constraint.

This book draws from ethnographic research conducted inside a New England state prison system and the surrounding community from 2011 to 2013. The setting is hereafter assigned the fictional name "Melville" in order to maintain the study participants' anonymity. The research comprised 77 semi-structured interviews and hundreds of hours of observation across seven correctional facilities ranging from minimum to supermax security. Participants in this research included short and long-term inmates, correctional healthcare providers, correctional officers, prison administrators, ex-inmates, families of inmates, and community-based physicians and social workers. An assortment of public and private peri-carceral spaces collectively comprised the research setting.

The prison was located atop a high hill, rolling up from a river, in an area known as the Melville reservation. Situated 10 miles southwest of a major New England city, the reservation has a university campus-like feel consisting of a series of Victorian stone structures, several twentieth-century colonial revival brick buildings, and an assortment of modern

[1]The Bureau of Justice Statistics defines jails as locally operated, short term facilities that hold inmates awaiting trial or sentencing or both, and inmates sentenced to a term of less than one year, typically misdemeanants. Prisons are long term facilities run by the state or the federal government and typically hold felons and inmates with sentences of more than one year (Bureau of Justice Statistics, 2015). This book uses the term "prison" when referring to the penal system more generally.

cinderblock structures completed between the 1970s and mid-1990s. The reservation was home to seven active penal facilities, which housed up to approximately 3800 offenders at any given moment. Also located on the reservation was the Melville State Sheriff's Department, adult Probation & Parole, the only state psychiatric hospital, correctional officer's union, and prison administrative buildings.

This book depicts the lives of inmates living with HIV and who passed through the Melville prison system during the course of research. In prison, this group had access to HIV and primary medical care, mental health services, dental care, addiction treatment, and integrated case management support linking persons in the correctional setting to the community. Upon release, inmates received continued case management services through community HIV services, primary medical care, addiction treatment, mental healthcare services, health insurance programmes, and other public assistance.

1.1 Who Is Behind Bars?

The U.S. incarcerates 2.2 million people at any given moment, making it the largest prisoner population in the world (Wagner & Sawyer, 2018). By comparison, other industrial nations imprison 5–7 times fewer people than the U.S. (Dyer, 2000). From the 1920s to the 1970s, the growth rate of U.S. incarceration remained relatively stable (National Research Council, 2014). However, in recent decades the number of people behind bars has quadrupled. This historical expansion of the prison system has led scholars to refer to the current period as the era of "mass incarceration" (Garland, 2001). Expansion of prisons can be attributed to strict sentencing guidelines developed during the late 1980s and 1990s (e.g., "get tough on crime", "war on drugs", "three strike policy", and mandatory minimum sentencing laws) (Butterfield, 2003; NAACP, 2015).

The prison population unduly draws from poor urban communities with limited access to health and social resources both before and after incarceration (Mallik-kane & Visher, 2008; Travis, 2000; Travis, Solomon, & Waul, 2001). Racially, the prison population is disproportionately comprised of Black men. In 2013, the Federal Bureau of

Justice Statistics reported that 526,000 African-American men did time in state and federal correctional facilities, representing 37% of the total prison population. Additionally, there were 1,157,000 African-American men on parole and probation during this time (Carson, 2013). Taken together, 1.68 million Black men were under some form of state or federal supervision (excluding local jails) during 2013, a figure that equates to over 800,000 more black men behind bars when compared to the number of Black men listed as "slaves" in the 1850 U.S. census (Mulvaney, 2014).

State inmates average less than eleven years of schooling, up to a third of inmates are unemployed upon entering prison, and the average wage of those who were employed at the time of their incarceration was lower than persons with the same level of education (Western & Wildeman, 2009). Imprisonment does not help people escape from poor community conditions but rather amplifies social and structural deprivation. Western & Pettit found that if a person serves any time behind bars, his hourly wage will decrease by approximately 11%, annual employment by nine weeks, and annual earnings by 40% (Western & Pettit, 2010). Further, incarceration has deep-seated collateral consequences that transcend localised community settings. For example, American epidemiologist Ernest Drucker found that 50% of people sent to prison from New York City came from fourteen neighbourhoods in the Bronx, Manhattan, and Brooklyn, neighbourhoods where only 17% of New York adults reside (Drucker, 2011). In turn, individuals left behind in the community experience fractured social ties, economic losses for dependents, increased divorce rates, and prolonged stress among family and friends. This condition has lasting intergenerational impacts on health and future criminal justice involvement (Barreras, Drucker, & Rosenthal, 2005).

The prison population experiences a high burden of communicable and non-communicable disease (Flanigan et al., 2009; Maruschak, Berzofsky, & Unangst, 2015), mental health challenges (James & Glaze, 2006), and alcohol and drug dependency (Chandler, Fletcher, Volkow, 2009; Charuvastra et al., 2001). Because of these factors, the prison has been identified as a vital space for delivering public health and safety

(Greifinger, Bick, & Goldenson, 2007). For example, inmates consistently demonstrate elevated HIV levels when compared with the general community (Massoglia & Remster, 2019). In the U.S., HIV is 5-times higher in prison than in the general population (Flanigan et al., 2009). Approximately 1.2 million persons living with HIV, one-sixth of all Americans living with this condition, will pass through the U.S. prison system at some point in their lives (Spaulding et al., 2009).

Over 95% of inmates will eventually leave the correctional setting (Hughes & Wilson, 2004). However, two-thirds of state prison inmates will be re-arrested for a new crime within three years of release, and three-quarters within five years of release (Durose, Cooper, & Snyder, 2014). Inmates leaving prison typically go from a highly structured environment to low-level or no supervision. Returning inmates are often immediately exposed to high-risk places, people, and situations, and few have developed the prevention skills during their incarceration to deal with a range of social, economic, and health risks they commonly encounter during the re-entry period (Mallik-kane & Visher, 2008; Travis et al., 2001). Inmates returning to the community report challenges re-establishing family connections, finding employment, receiving healthcare, and dealing with finances (Travis et al., 2001). All of these factors contribute to a high likelihood of inmate recidivism and greatly jeopardise community health and safety (Clear, 2007; Freaudenberg, 2005; Lincoln, Miles, & Scheibel, 2007; Mallik-kane & Visher, 2008; Travis et al., 2001).

1.2 Prison Healthcare

Prison healthcare models vary from state-to-state and across healthcare providers. In theory, imprisonment offers improved access to medical attention when compared with many community settings (Greifinger et al., 2007). Currently, imprisonment is the only space where Americans have a constitutional right to healthcare ("Estelle v. Gamble, 429 U.S. 97", 1976). While imprisonment intends to deliver "equal access" medical care, the reality is complex and often enables only negligible care and treatment (Allen, Wakeman, Cohen, & Rich, 2010; Thompson, 2010).

The Estelle v. Gamble ruling entitles inmates to a professional medical judgement, diagnosis, and treatment access. It calls any disallowance of medical care in prison to be a "deliberate indifference to serious medical needs", and thus in violation of the Eighth Amendment of the U.S. Constitution. However, the ruling's precise wording has led to a high threshold in defining "serious medical need", leading some inmates to self-harm to draw attention from medical staff (Thompson, 2010). Equally, "deliberate indifference" sets a low standard of medical care provision, where inmates are not protected from insufficient treatment stemming from an "accident, inadvertent behaviour, or ordinary negligence" (Thompson, 2010, p. 638).

Many inmates with physical and mental illness do not receive adequate treatment in prison, and medical treatment rates further decline after inmates return to the community. A widely cited 2008 study of prison leavers in Ohio and Texas found that two-thirds of men and three-quarters of women with physical health conditions received treatment in prison, a percentage that fell to one-half of men and six in ten women at eight to ten months after they returned to the general community. The study also reports similar patterns for the treatment of mental illness and substance addiction (Mallik-kane & Visher, 2008).

1.3 HIV Policy and Care

While HIV prevalence in correctional settings has decreased since the late 1990s, an increase in the size of the incarcerated population has resulted in a consistent number of HIV cases in prisons and jails (Spaulding et al., 2009). This current state has been described as a persistent HIV epidemic (Westergaard, Spaulding, & Flanigan, 2013). Clark, Stine, Hanna, Sobota, and Rich (2001) and Hammett (2006) describe high-risk sexual behaviour, injection drug use, and tattooing as contributing factors for HIV, hepatitis, and other STI transmission within correctional settings. Most new infections within prison have been linked to male-to-male sex and tattooing practices (Centers for Disease Control and Prevention, 2006; Jafa et al., 2009). However, Beckwith, Zaller, Fu, Montague and Rich (2010) identify how research findings on the prevalence of HIV-transmission within prisons vary across settings. For example, a study in the Georgia Department of Corrections found that 88 new HIV infections occurred within prison from 1992 to 2005. Around the same time, another study in the Rhode Island Department of Corrections followed 587 inmates for 12 months and found that all participants were HIV-negative at baseline, and none of these individuals seroconverted during a 12-month observation period (Macalino et al., 2004). While Hammett (2006) highlights a real risk for infections occurring within the prison setting, Beckwith et al. (2010) claim that a majority of HIV transmission occurs in the public community before a person's incarceration.

Given the large number of people living with HIV who pass through prisons and jails, there has been increased recognition that the criminal justice system should serve as an intervention point for identifying and linking persons with HIV into care and treatment. The Centers for Disease Control and Prevention (CDC) has called for routine adult HIV testing since 2006 (Branson et al., 2006; CDC, 2009). However, due to logistical challenges, described in previous reviews (Beckwith et al., 2010; Flanigan et al., 2010), adequate testing practices are still underutilised in over half of all correctional facilities nationally (Westergaard et al., 2013).

Not all HIV-positive persons will require immediate treatment upon becoming incarcerated, but all should have appropriate screening and regular laboratory testing. Highly active antiviral therapy (HAART) has been shown to most effectively treat HIV-positive individuals and decrease the incidence of opportunistic infections and AIDS-related mortality (Beckwith et al., 2010). However, a 2005 national survey of correctional facilities reported that 59% of city and county jails and 71% of state and federal prisons provided HAART to inmates with

CD4 counts[2] of 300 or higher[3] (Hammett, Kennedy, & Kuck, 2007). Although, a later study in 2007 estimated far bleaker statistics, reporting that only 33% of inmates with HIV receive HAART in the U.S. correctional setting (Zaller, Thurmond, & Rich, 2007). Both studies highlight a range of treatment standards and non-consensus on when it is appropriate to commence antiviral therapy for HIV-positive inmates.

There are several obstacles to delivering antiviral treatment in the correctional setting. Challenges specific to corrections arise over the loss of confidentiality because many HIV-positive inmates are placed in separate housing, are seen by specific medical staff, and have their status easily identified through other mechanisms (Earnshaw & Chaudoir, 2009). Medication dispensing protocols also create barriers to treatment adherence, and inmates often experience treatment disruptions when transferring facilities (Belenko, 2013).

1.4 Community Re-Entry and HIV Support

Over 12 million people (representing 9 million individual cases) pass through U.S. jails each year (Ramaswamy & Freaudenberg, 2007). Additionally, some 600,000 inmates will leave state and federal prisons annually, equating to about 1600 prison leavers every day (Hughes & Wilson, 2004; Travis et al., 2001). Many inmates leaving prison remain under some level of state supervision, a status known as "community-based corrections" or "parole". At year-end 2013, an estimated 4,751,400 ex-inmates were on active parole (Herberman & Bonczar, 2014).

Persons leaving prison will often go from a highly structured environment to low-level or no supervision. Upon leaving prison, people face challenges, including access to food, housing, social integration, and legal and parole conditions (Rich et al., 2013). This transitional time has also

[2]Cluster of differentiation 4 (CD4) is a surrogate biological marker to determine an HIV-positive persons response to antiretroviral treatment (Egger et al., 2002; Mellors et al., 1997).

[3]The U.S. Department of Health and Human Services and the International Antiviral Society guidelines for HIV treatment recommend antiretroviral treatment be provided to all HIV-positive persons, regardless of CD4 cell counts. Other clinical advisory groups such as the British HIV Association and the European AIDS Clinical Society offer alternative guidance for antiviral therapy (Lundgren, Babiker, Gordin, Borges, & Neaton, 2013).

been associated with a heightened risk of mortality. One study in Washington State found that the risk of mortality among former inmates was 12.7 times higher during the two weeks after an inmate leaves prison when compared to other members of the community (Binswanger et al., 2007). The leading causes of death among returning inmates include drug overdose, cardiovascular disease, homicide, and suicide (Binswanger et al., 2007).

Support offered to inmates leaving a carceral setting is often minimal. Only 10% of persons leaving prison received discharge planning, a percentage of prison leavers that have shrunk over recent decades (Dumont, Kuester, & Rich, 2014; Mellow & Greifinger, 2005; Travis et al., 2001). Nevertheless, there is a growing effort from a range of individuals, including medical practitioners, public health professionals, and government organisations to develop comprehensive discharge planning and re-entry support. Some have referred to this movement as an emerging "re-entry industry" (Thompkins, 2010).

Current prisoner re-entry programmes are typically divided into three phases: programmes that work with inmates within prison, programmes that connect ex-inmates to services during release, and programmes that provide sustained support and supervision after inmates transition to life in the community. Most inmate re-entry programmes focus on health and involve multi-sector collaborations. For example, in Massachusetts, Hampden County Jail has coordinated support between the county sheriff's office, public health department, local medical centres, and public health centres to provide discharge planning, case management services, and healthcare delivery for inmates leaving regional jails. While evaluations of this programme remain incomplete, they do indicate some improved inmate and community health, decreased recidivism, and cost savings (Conklin, Lincoln, & Wilson, 2002).

Since 1990, there have been three major community-based public payers of HIV care for returning inmates, including the federal-funded Medicare, federal- and state-funded Medicaid entitlement programmes, and the discretionary Ryan White HIV/AIDS Program (AIDS Drugs Assistance Program (ADAP)). These programmes have remained critical to the Affordable Care Act (ACA) today (Montague et al., 2012). The ACA provides new opportunities to address low insurance coverage rates among newly released offenders (Bandara et al. 2015). However, Medicaid has a longstanding policy of excluding coverage to those who are incarcerated, a policy that remains under the ACA (Department of Health & Human Services, 2016). Nevertheless, this changing healthcare landscape has led to some states adopting policies to suspend rather than terminate coverage as a measure to improve continuity of care for released inmates (Medicaid and CHIP Payment and Access Commission, 2018). That said, delays in lifting suspended coverage persist due to communication failures between Medicare Services and the prison system and challenges with patient record sharing (Department of Health & Human Services, 2016). Persons who have their coverage terminated while incarcerated face substantial delays and reapplication. Consequently, prisoners who received Medicaid before imprisonment often lack this health insurance on release. Similarly, disenrollment practices for Social Security Income (SSI) and Social Security Disability Income (SSDI) result in returning offenders suffering without benefits for months or longer, exacerbating financial challenges for those unable to work (Wakeman, McKinney, & Rich, 2009).

Among people living with HIV, formerly incarcerated persons have a higher prevalence of mental illness, substance use, and homelessness, making their transition back into the community incredibly daunting (Haley et al., 2014; Springer & Altice, 2007; Travis et al., 2001). Since 1996, case management interventions to facilitate connections between correctional-based and community-based resources have been developed in settings for HIV re-entry support (Petersilia, 2003; Rich et al., 2001; Westergaard et al., 2013). Previous evaluations provide details of these programmes (Draine, 2011; Springer, Spaulding, Meyer, & Altice, 2011).

Evidence of the achievements of case management programmes remains mixed. Numerous studies demonstrate short-term benefits to linking individuals into care through case management (Avery, Ciomica, Gierlach, & Machekano, 2019; Baillargeon et al., 2009; Gardner et al., 2005). However, a highly cited randomised control trial observed no significant difference between case management and standard discharge release programmes on critical health outcomes, including immediate linkage to care (Wohl, 2011). Other observational studies have shown similar ineffectual results (Arriola, Braithwaite, Holmes, & Fortenberry, 2007; Murphree, Batey, Kay, Westfall, & Mugavero, 2019), and one study demonstrates that case management has no long-term care effects (Miller, Chiaramonte, Mcnall, Forney, & Janulis, 2018).

1.5 Does Violence Lead to Health?

Prison is not a neutral or taken-for-granted space but is revealing of, and constituted within, the context in which it is situated. This book's introduction highlights a myriad of structural deprivations and public health challenges underpinning inmates' lived experience of HIV. This book will shed light on what initially seemed to be a curious research finding: Many people living with HIV use violence to improve their health and wellbeing. Violence, which for some included the act of becoming imprisoned, facilitated a unique claims-making process against the state by affording HIV-positive people with offending histories access to resources and rights that were otherwise unattainable.

Research participants referred to this violence as "degradation". This encompassed a routinised production and consumption of "*abjectionable*", illicit, or "un-citizenly" behaviour for the pursuit of rights and resources in relationship with prison staff. It had long-lasting effects in terms of generating agency and livelihood for criminal justice-involved persons living with HIV, yet at the same time propelling them into conditions of subjugation through continually lowering their dignity, character, social standing, and physical wellbeing.

This book interrogates the notion of degradation as a delicately balanced mechanism for the pursuit of health. I will draw on multiple accounts to explore how degradation is produced, consumed, and understood by inmates and prison staff as inmates move from prison to the community. This book examines several questions: where and in what form "agency" takes within a context of exceptional violence and constraint?; How do inmates and staff engage in tasks of daily living within a shared space of imprisonment?; What might be considered "degrading", and how is it used and understood within prison?; How are security, medical, prisoner re-entry, and welfare organisations complicit in practices of degradation and how is degradation co-produced and mirrored by other individuals within the prison system, as well as sustained at the level of face-to-face interactions between staff and inmates?

Chapter 2 positions this research within a tradition of American prison ethnography. This chapter draws attention to an emerging idea of "productive violence" as a critical lens from which to understand the theoretical development of degradation, a concept accounting for the social and physical violence observed in Melville prison. I will describe the methodology and methods underpinning the ethnographic research informing this book. This will include describing access to the research field, data generation, and analytical treatment of data. This chapter will also outline the ethical challenges encountered during research.

Chapter 3 introduces the concept of "degradation" and how it is practiced through "prison games", an interactive process between inmates and prison staff. It describes how degradation is necessary for inmates' agency, the ability to create change, and, ultimately, their survival.

Chapter 4 details the benefits of prison games for inmates. It outlines what can be gained as situationally determined, delicately balanced outcomes in relation to more deleterious effects. I will highlight how degradation allows a person to exploit and move between criminal and ill identities. This chapter will move beyond discussing how inmates engage in prison games to access medical care and provide a more nuanced examination of how inmates go about playing prison games in order to gain access to a range of rights and resources.

Chapter 5 turns attention to the prison staff involved in the playing of prison games. Staff understand and manage prison games in relation to their social world inside the prison and outside in the community. While staff try to present themselves as socially distinct from inmates, they also have biographical experiences in common. Therefore, I explore how staff, like inmates, become enmeshed in prison violence. This chapter proceeds in three steps. First, it explores how staff have similar biographical histories in the community and a shared experience of "doing time" together. Both inmates and staff expressed dependence on the prison to maintain or advance their social positions. Next, this chapter describes a staff work culture, training practices, and supervision that contribute to the playing of prison games. Finally, this chapter will explain staff performance of wealth and acts of degradation as a means of establishing inmates as socially different from themselves.

Chapter 6 will continue to explore the experience of prison games from the perspective of staff. In this chapter, I describe the process whereby staff are included in playing prison games over time. Staff sees themselves as not mattering positively in their professional role, which was defined by a punishment culture. This chapter describes how staff participation in prison games is socially policed and highlights how some staff still enact subtle moments of care within a violent context. This chapter shows how, in a context imbued with violence, no one is immune to its effects.

This book concludes by outlining the theoretical development of degradation and prison games. I will consider research findings alongside other scholarly work on prison violence. Further, I will look at other global models of imprisonment to suggest how institutional reforms for offenders and staff might be made to address the use and production of violence among HIV-positive inmates in the U.S. prison context.

References

Allen, S. A., Wakeman, S. E., Cohen, R. L., & Rich, D. J. (2010). Physicians in US prisons in the era of mass incarceration. *International Journal of Prison Health, 6*(3), 100–106.

Arriola, K. R. J., Braithwaite, R. L., Holmes, N. E., & Fortenberry, R. M. (2007). Post-release case management services and health-seeking behavior among HIV-infected ex-offenders. *Journal of Health Care for the Poor and Underserved, 18*(3), 665–674.

Avery, A., Ciomica, R., Gierlach, M., & Machekano, R. (2019). Jail-based case management improves retention in HIV care 12 months post release. *AIDS and Behavior, 23*(4), 966–972.

Baillargeon, J., Giordano, T. P., Rich, J. D., Wu, Z. H., Wells, K., Pollock, B. H., & Paar, D. P. (2009). Accessing antiretroviral therapy following release from prison. *Journal of the American Medical Association, 301*(8), 848–857.

Bandara, S. N., Huskamp, H. A., Riedel, L. E., McGinty, E. E., Webster, D., Toone, R. E., & Barry, C. L. (2015). Leveraging the affordable care act to enroll justice-involved populations in medicaid: State and local efforts. *Health Affairs, 34*(12), 2044–2051.
Barreras, R. E., Drucker, E. M., & Rosenthal, D. (2005). The concentration of substance use, criminal justice involvement, and HIV/AIDS in the families of drug offenders. *Journal of Urban Health, 82*(1), 162–170.
Beckwith, C. G., Zaller, N. D., Fu, J. J., Montague, B. T., & Rich, J. D. (2010). Opportunities to diagnose, treat, and prevent HIV in the criminal justice system. *Journal of Acquired Immune Deficiency Syndromes, 55*(Suppl 1), S49–S55.
Belenko, S., Hiller, M., Visher, C., Copenhaver, M., O'Connell, D., Burdon, W., Pankow, J., Clarke, J., & Oser, C. (2013). Policies and practices in the delivery of HIV services in correctional agencies and facilities: Results from a multi-site survey. *Journal of Correctional Health Care, 19*(4), 293–310.
Binswanger, I. A., Stern, M. F., Deyo, R. A., Heagerty, P. J., Cheadle, A., Elmore, J. G., & Koepsell, T. D. (2007). Release from prison–A high risk of death for former inmates. *The New England Journal of Medicine, 356*(2), 157–165.
Branson, B. M., Handsfield, H. H., Lampe, M. A., Janssen, R. S., Taylor, A. W., Lyss, S. B., & Clark, J. E. (2006). Revised recommendations for HIV testing of adults, adolescents, and pregnant women in health-care settings. *MMWR Recommendations and Reports, 55*(14), 1–17.
Bureau of Justice Statistics. (2015). *FAQ Detail, What is the difference between jails and prisons?* Retrieved from http://www.bjs.gov/index.cfm?ty=qa&iid=322.
Butterfield, F. (2003, July 28). Study finds 2.6% increase in U.S. prisoner population. *New York Times*. Retrieved from http://www.nytimes.com/2003/07/28/us/study-finds-2.6-increase-in-us-prison-population.html.
Carson, E. A. (2013). *Prisoners in 2013*. Washington, DC. Retrieved from http://www.bjs.gov/content/pub/pdf/p.13.pdf.
Center for Disease Control and Prevention. (2009). *HIV testing implementation guidance for correctional settings*. Retrieved from https://stacks.cdc.gov/view/cdc/5279/cdc_5279_DS1.pdf.
Centers for Disease Control and Prevention. (2006). HIV transmission among male inmates in a state prison system—Georgia, 1992–2005. *Morbidity and Mortality Weekly Report (MMWR), 55*(15), 421–426. Retrieved from http://www.cdc.gov/mmwr/preview/mmwrhtml/mm5515a1.htm.

Chandler, R. K., Fletcher, B. W., & Volkow, N. D. (2009). Treating drug abuse and addiction in the criminal justice system: Improving public health and safety. *Journal of the American Medical Association, 301*(2), 183–190.
Charuvastra, A., Stein, J., Schwartzapfel, B., Spaulding, A., Horowitz, E., Macalino, G., & Rich, J. D. (2001). Hepatitis B vaccination practices in state and federal prisons. *Public Health Reports, 116*(3), 203–209.
Clarke, J. G., Stine, M. D., Hanna, L., Sobota, M., & Rich, D. J. (2001). Active and former injection drug users report of HIV risk behaviors during periods of incarceration. *Substance Abuse, 22*(4), 209–216.
Clear, T. R. (2007). Impact of incarceration on community public safety and public health. In R. B. Greifinger, J. A. Bick, & J. Goldenson (Eds.), *Public Health Behind Bars, From Prisons to Communities* (pp. 13–24). New York, NY: Springer.
Conklin, T., Lincoln, T., & Wilson, R. (2002). *A public health manual for correctional health care*. Hampden County Sheriff's Department and Massachusetts Public Health Association: Ludlow, MA. Retrieved from https://www.prearesourcecenter.org/sites/default/files/library/phmodelforcorrectionalhealth.pdf.
Department of Health & Human Services. (2016). *To facilitate sucessful re-entry for individuals transitioning from incarceration to their communities; The state health offical letter.* Retrieved from https://www.medicaid.gov/federal-policy-guidance/downloads/sho16007.pdf.
Draine, J., Ahuja, D., Altice, F. L., Arriola, K. J., Avery, A. K., Beckwith, C., Booker, C. A., … Tinsley, M. J. (2011). Strategies to enhance linkages between care for HIV/AIDS in jail and community settings. *AIDS Care, 23*(3), 366–377.
Drucker, E. (2011). *A plague of prisons: The epidemiology of mass incarceration in America*. New York, NY: The New Press.
Dumont, D. M., Kuester, L. B., & Rich, D. J. (2014). Health issues in prison reentry models. In G. Bruinsma & D. Weisburd (Eds.), *Encyclopedia of criminology and criminal justice* (pp. 2053–2062). New York, NY: Springer.
Durose, M. R., Cooper, A. D., & Snyder, H. N. (2014). *Recidivism of prisoners released in 30 states in 2005: Patterns from 2005 to 2012*. Bureau of Justice Statistics: Washington, DC. Retrieved from http://www.bjs.gov/index.cfm?ty=pbdetail&iid=4986.
Dyer, J. (2000). *The perpetual prisoner machine: How America profits from crime*. Boulder, CO: Westview Press.

Earnshaw, V. A., & Chaudoir, S. R. (2009). From conceptualizing to measuring HIV stigma: A review of HIV stigma mechanism measures. *AIDS and Behavior, 13*(6), 1160–1177.

Egger, M., May, M., Chene, G., Phillips, A. N., Ledergerber, B., Dabis, F.,… Sterne, J. A. (2002). Prognosis of HIV-1-infected patients starting highly active antiretroviral therapy: A collaborative analysis of prospective studies. *Lancet, 360*(9327), 119–129. Retrieved from http://www.ncbi.nlm.nih.gov/pubmed/12126821.

Estelle v. Gamble, 429 U.S. 97, 97 426 (Supreme Court of the United States 1976).

Flanigan, T. P., Zaller, N., Beckwith, C. G., Bazerman, L. B., Rana, A., Gardner, A., … Altice, F. L. (2010). Testing for HIV, sexually transmitted infections, and viral hepatitis in jails: still a missed opportunity for public health and HIV prevention. *Journal of Acquired Immune Deficiency Syndromes, 55 Suppl 2*, S78–83.

Flanigan, T. P., Zaller, N., Taylor, L., Beckwith, C., Kuester, L., Rich, J., & Carpenter, C. C. (2009). HIV and infectious disease care in jails and prisons: breaking down the walls with the help of academic medicine. *Transactions of the American Clinical and Climatological Association, 120*, 73–83.

Freaudenberg, N. (2005). Coming home from jail: The social and health consequences of community reentry for women, male adolescents, and their families and communities. *American Journal of Public Health, 95*(10).

Gardner, L. I., Metsch, L. R., Anderson-Mahoney, P., Loughlin, A. M., del Rio, C., Strathdee, S., Sansom, S. L., … Holmberg, S. D. (2005). Efficacy of a brief case management intervention to link recently diagnosed HIV-infected persons to care. *AIDS, 19*(4), 423–431.

Garland, D. (2001). *Mass imprisonment social causes and consequences* (pp. 1 online resource (vii, 184 p.)). Retrieved from http://knowledge.sagepub.com/view/mass-imprisonment/SAGE.xml.

Greifinger, R. B., Bick, J. A., & Goldenson, J. (2007). *Public health behind bars: From prisons to communities*. New York, NY: Springer.

Haley, D. F., Golin, C. E., Farel, C. E., Wohl, D. A., Scheyett, A. M., Garrett, J. J., Rosen, D. L., & Parker, S. D. (2014). Multilevel challenges to engagement in HIV care after prison release: a theory-informed qualitative study comparing prisoners' perspectives before and after community reentry. *BMC Public Health, 14*, 1253.

Hammet, T. M. (2006). HIV/AIDS and other infectious diseases among correctional inmates: Transmission, burden, and appropriate response. *American Journal of Public Health, 96*(6), 974–978.
Hammett, T. M., Kennedy, S., & Kuck, S. (2007). *National survey of infectious diseases in correctional facilities: HIV and sexually transmitted diseases.* Retrieved from https://www.ncjrs.gov/pdffiles1/nij/grants/217736.pdf.
Herberman, E. J., & Bonczar, T. P. (2014). *Probation and parole in the United States, 2013.* Bureau of Justice Statistics: Washington, DC: Retrieved from http://www.bjs.gov/index.cfm?ty=pbdetail&iid=5135.
Hughes, T., & Wilson, D. J. (2004). *Reentry trends in the United States: Inmates returning to the community after serving time in prison.* Bureau of Justice Statistics: Washington, DC. Retrieved from http://www.bjs.gov/content/pub/pdf/reentry.pdf.
Jafa, K., McElroy, P., Fitzpatrick, L., Borkowf, C. B., Macgowan, R., Margolis, A., … Sullivan, P. S. (2009). HIV transmission in a state prison system, 1988-2005. *Plos One, 4*(5), e5416.
James, D. J., & Glaze, L. E. (2006). *Special report: Mental health problems of prison and jail inmates.* Retrieved from http://www.ojp.usdoj.gov/bjs/abstract/mhppji.htm.
Lincoln, T., Miles, J. R., & Scheibel, S. (2007). Community health and public health collaborations. In R. B. Greifinger, J. A. Bick, & J. Goldenson (Eds.), *Public helath behind bars: From prisons to communities.* New York, NY: Springer.
Lundgren, J. D., Babiker, A. G., Gordin, F. M., Borges, A. H., & Neaton, J. D. (2013). When to start antiretroviral therapy: The need for an evidence base during early HIV infection. *BMC Medicine, 11*(148), 1–10. Retrieved from http://www.biomedcentral.com/content/pdf/1741-7015-11-148.pdf.
Macalino, G. E., Vlahov, D., Sanford-Colby, S., Patel, S., Sabin, K., Salas, C., & Rich, J. D. (2004). Prevalence and incidence of HIV, hepatitis B virus, and hepatitis C virus infections among males in Rhode Island prisons. *American Journal of Public Health, 94*(7), 1218–1223. Retrieved from http://www.ncbi.nlm.nih.gov/pubmed/15226146.
Mallik-kane, K., & Visher, C. A. (2008). *Health and prisoner reentry: How physical, mental, and substance abuse conditions shape the process of reintegration.* Urban Institute, Justice Policy Center: Washington, DC. Retrieved from https://www.urban.org/sites/default/files/publication/31491/411617-Health-and-Prisoner-Reentry.PDF.
Maruschak, L. M., Berzofsky, M., & Unangst, J. (2015). *Medical problems of state and federal prisoners and jail inmates, 2011–2012.* U.S. Department of

Justice, Bureau of Justice Statistics: Washington, DC. Retrieved from https://www.bjs.gov/content/pub/pdf/mpsfpji1112.pdf.

Massoglia, M., & Remster, B. (2019). Linkages between incarceration and health. *Public Health Reports, 134,* 8s–14s.

Medicaid and CHIP Payment and Access Commission. (2018). *Medicaid and the criminal justice system.* Retrieved from https://www.macpac.gov/wp-content/uploads/2018/07/Medicaid-and-the-Criminal-Justice-System.pdf.

Mellors, J. W., Munoz, A., Giorgi, J. V., Margolick, J. B., Tassoni, C. J., Gupta, P.,… Rinaldo, C. R., Jr. (1997). Plasma viral load and CD4 + lymphocytes as prognostic markers of HIV-1 infection. *Annals of Internal Medicine, 126*(12), 946–954. Retrieved from http://www.ncbi.nlm.nih.gov/pubmed/9182471.

Mellow, J., & Greifinger, R. B. (2005). Successful reentry: The perspective of private correctional health care providers. *Journal of Urban Health, 84,* 85–98.

Miller, R. L., Chiaramonte, D., Mcnall, M. A., Forney, J. C., & Janulis, P. F. (2018). Living with HIV after release from prison: An evaluation of the long-term health of formerly incarcerated individuals who used Michigan's Community Reentry Service. *Journal of Prison Education and Reentry, 5*(2), 171–184.

Montague, B. T., Rosen, D. L., Solomon, L., Nunn, A., Green, T., Costa, M., … Rich, J. D. (2012). Tracking linkage to HIV care for former prisoners: A public health priority. *Virulence, 3*(3), 319–324.

Mulvaney, K. (2014, December 7th). Brow U. student leader: More African American men in prison system now than were enslaved in 1850. *Providence Journal.* Retrieved from http://www.politifact.com/rhode-island/statements/2014/dec/07/diego-arene-morley/brown-u-student-leader-more-african-american-men-p/.

Murphree, J., Batey, D. S., Kay, E. S., Westfall, A. O., & Mugavero, M. J. (2019). Suboptimal retention in care among recently released rrisoners: Implications for social workers in HIV primary care. *AIDS and Behavior, 23*(2), 427–432.

NAACP. (2015). *Criminal justice fact sheet.* Retrieved from http://www.naacp.org/pages/criminal-justice-fact-sheet.

National Research Council. (2014). *The growth of incarceration in the United States, exploring causes and consequences.* Retrieved from https://johnjay.jjay.cuny.edu/nrc/NAS_report_on_incarceration.pdf.

Petersilia, J. (2003). *When prisoners come home: Parole and prisoner reentry.* Oxford and New York: Oxford University Press.

Ramaswamy, M., & Freaudenberg, N. (2007). Health promotion in jails and prisons: an alternative paradigm for correctional health services. In R. B. Greifinger (Ed.), *Public health behind bars: From prisons to communities*. New York, NY: Springer.

Rich, J. D., DiClemente, R., Levy, J., Lyda, K., Ruiz, M. S., Rosen, D. L., & Dumont, D. (2013). Correctional facilities as partners in reducing HIV disparities. *Jaids-Journal of Acquired Immune Deficiency Syndromes, 63*, S49–S53.

Rich, J. D., Holmes, L., Salas, C., Macalino, G., Davis, D., Ryczek, J., & Flanigan, T. (2001). Successful linkage of medical care and community services for HIV-positive offenders being released from prison. *Journal Urban Health, 78*(2), 279–289.

Spaulding, A. C., Seals, R. M., Page, M. J., Brzozowski, A. K., Rhodes, W., & Hammett, T. M. (2009). HIV/AIDS among inmates of and releasees from US correctional facilities, 2006: Declining share of epidemic but persistent public health opportunity. *Plos One, 4*(11), A16–A21.

Springer, S. A., & Altice, F. L. (2007). Improving the care for HIV-infected prisoners: An integrated Prison-release health model. In R. B. Greifinger (Ed.), *Public health behind bars: From prisons to communities* (pp. 535–555). New York, NY: Springer.

Springer, S. A., Spaulding, A. C., Meyer, J. P., & Altice, F. L. (2011). Public health implications for adequate transitional care for HIV-infected prisoners: Five essential components. *Clinical Infectious Diseases, 53*, 469–479.

Thompkins, D. E. (2010). The expanding prisoner reentry industry. *Dialectical Anthropology, 34*, 589–604.

Thompson, J. H. (2010). Today's deliberate indifference: Providing attention without providing treatment to prisoners with serious medical needs. *Harvard Civil Rights-Civil Liberties Law Review, 45*(2), 635–654.

Travis, J. (2000). *But they all come back: Rethinking prisoner reentry*. National Institute of Justice: Washington, DC. Retrieved from https://www.ncjrs.gov/pdffiles1/nij/181413.pdf.

Travis, J., Solomon, A. L., & Waul, M. (2001). *From prison to home: The dimensions and consequences of prisoner reentry*. Urban Institute, Justice Policy Center: Washington, DC. Retrieved from https://www.urban.org/sites/default/files/publication/61571/410098-From-Prison-to-Home-The-Dimensions-and-Consequences-of-Prisoner-Reentry.PDF.

Wagner, P., & Sawyer, W. (2018). *Mass incarceration: The whole pie 2018*. Retrieved from https://www.prisonpolicy.org/reports/pie2018.html.

Wakeman, S. E., McKinney, M. E., & Rich, J. D. (2009). Filling the gap: The importance of medicaid continuity for former inmates. *Journal of General Internal Medicine, 24*(7), 860–862.
Westergaard, R. P., Spaulding, A. C., & Flanigan, T. P. (2013). HIV among persons incarcerated in the USA: A review of evolving concepts in testing, treatment, and linkage to community care. *Current Opinion in Infectious Diseases, 26*(1), 10–16.
Western, B., & Pettit, B. (2010). *Collateral costs: Incarceration's effect on economic mobility*. The Pew Charitable Trusts: Washington DC: Retrieved from https://www.pewtrusts.org/~/media/legacy/uploadedfiles/pcs_assets/2010/collateralcosts1pdf.pdf.
Western, B., & Wildeman, C. (2009). The black family and mass incarceration. *Annals of the American Academy of Political and Social Science, 621*, 221–242.
Wohl, D. A., Scheyett, A., Golin, C. E., White, B., Matuszewski, J., Bowling, M., Smith, P., … Earp, J. (2011). Intensive case management before and after prison release is no more effective than comprehensive pre-release discharge planning in linking HIV-infected prisoners to care: A randomized trial. *AIDS and Behavior, 15*(2), 356–364.
Zaller, N., Thurmond, P., & Rich, D. J. (2007). Limited spending: An analysis of correctional expenditures on antiretrovirals for HIV-infected prisoners. *Public Health Reports, 122*(1), 49–54.

2

A Study on Prison Violence and HIV

2.1 American Prison Ethnography

American prison ethnography has eclipsed in recent decades, while Europe and other regions have observed a resurgence in this type of research (Cunha, 2014; Rhodes, 2001; Wacquant, 2002). Comparing international ethnographic findings builds a greater understanding of prison culture, however, U.S. institutions have their own values, politics, and orthodoxies that shape the experience of imprisonment and HIV. Therefore, it is worth highlighting the research trajectory and gaps within the U.S. context.

The U.S. has a rich tradition of prison ethnography dating back to Donald Clemmer (1940) and Gresham Sykes (1958). Early descriptions render prison as a site where people are socially re-coded in isolation from mainstream society. In the 1960s, ethnographers moved away from depicting prisons as homogenous "small societies" or "societies of captives", and instead engaged in new explorations of external factors influencing prison cultures, proposing an "importation model" (Irwin, 1970, 1980, 1985; Irwin & Cressey, 1962). More recent ethnographies have focused on race and ethnicity (Carroll, 1974; Diaz-Cotto,

L. Kuester, *Violence in Pursuit of Health*, Palgrave Studies in Prisons and Penology, https://doi.org/10.1007/978-3-030-61350-1_2

1996; Wacquant, 2013); brutality, violence and social control (Colvin, 1992; Fleisher, 1989; Trammell, 2012), and gender (Kruttschnitt & Gartner, 2005; McCorkel, 2003; Owen, 1998; Ward & Kassebaum, 1965). Ethnographic studies have also included correctional officers (Crouch, 1980; Jacobs, 1977; Marquart, 1986; Philliber, 1987; Zimmer, 1986), healthcare staff (Rhodes, 2004), and family and social networks of inmates (Braman, 2007; Clear, Rose, & Ryder, 2001; Clear, 2007; Comfort, 2008).

Only a few international ethnographic studies have accounted for people living with HIV in prison. Research demonstrates that inmates were reluctant to disclose their HIV status upon entering the correctional setting, and inmates experienced challenges accessing treatment because of failures in stockpiling medication, confiscation of medication by security staff, and strikes (Esposito, 2012; Small, Wood, Betteridge, Montaner, & Kerr, 2009). A study of community re-entry programmes found that HIV-positive inmates transition to the community improved alongside rapport with case-managers and healthcare staff prior to their release (Nunn et al., 2010). Another prison-to-community study observed that while inmates initially optimistic about continuing HIV treatment before leaving prison, community follow-up highlighted multiple challenges related to stigma, substance use, housing, and finance (Haley et al., 2014).

This book depicts the experiences of people living with HIV as they move from prison to the community. It takes a whole systems approach, soliciting accounts from persons across social stratum and sampling all state prison facilities and an offender re-entry support programme. This book contributes to a new theorisation of violence within a prison context quintessentially marked by remarkable conditions of constraint.

2.2 Violence

"Violence" is an elusive concept addressing physical acts (hard violence) and social patterns (soft violence) that intersect with economic and political forces (Colaguori, 2010; Hann, 2008). Four distinct forms and expressions of violence have traditionally been captured in ethnographic research. These include "direct political violence" or physical violence and terror administered by authorities and those challenging it; "structural violence" or habitual, historically enriched political-economic oppression and social inequality, which might include exploitative international terms of trade and abusive working conditions; "symbolic violence" or internalised humiliations and legitimations of inequality and hierarchy ranging from sexism and racism to expressions of class power, and "everyday violence" or the daily practices and expressions of violence which focus on the individual experience normalising petty brutalities and terror at the community-level (Bourgois, 2001, p. 8).

Further, the study of "social suffering" offers a conceptual lens to understand how a person's everyday pains, miseries, and experiences of violence are caused and conditioned by society (Wilkinson, 2013). Social suffering can affect people across the social stratum, including those with ostensibly more power, but grind most brutally on the poor (Kleinman, 2000). Furthermore, violence is not limited by the act or interaction itself, as it can be present in "witnessing" and "memory" and how experiences are recollected can have trace effects in people's lives and social relationships (Das, 2000).

Ethnographic studies on violence and social suffering have traditionally focused on the viewpoints of persons and communities in distress, often neglecting to capture those with ostensibly more power within individual relationships and collective systems. Further, they often propagate the understanding that violence is categorically "destructive and evil" (Colaguori, 2010; Jauregui, 2013), missing opportunities to explore how violence can also become constructive and empowering for persons. Prison offers a chance to identify the agentic qualities that violence can create.

2.3 Violence in Prison

The act of violence invests the body with agency, not only the body of the perpetrator but also that of the victim and the survivor (Das, 1996). In prison, violence is both productive and destructive, and no one is immune to its effects. Criminologists writing about violence recognise that it has agentic qualities. For example, Edgar, O'Donnell and Martin

(2003) describe violence, while fundamentally harmful to people, is an act of rebellion against imposed order, and thus becomes necessary to redefine or renegotiate relationships (Edgar et al., 2003). These authors highlight how violence in this context might serve as a form of communication, taking on a different meaning within prison (Edgar et al., 2003, p. 9). Jauregui (2013) recognise the experience of agency that exists when examining police brutality, explaining violent behaviour blurs the categorical lines between the powerful and powerless, predicator and victim and oppressor and oppressed when its use is justified to uphold public order and safety. She highlights important epistemological and ontological problems for ethnographers who study violence, questioning "When, how, and for whom does violence, as a context, a social act or event, or an institutionalised process, become 'necessary' or'legitimate'? Who decides which boundary lines mark necessity, truth, and justice, and on what grounds?" (Jauregui, 2013, p. 129).

This book focuses on prison members' use of everyday acts considered to be disgusting and destructive (e.g., self-amputation of digits, urinating, or spitting). Actions recognised for their production of "*abjection*" (e.g., experiencing repulsion after being spat on) (Kristeva, 1982). The concept of *abjection* captures a psychosomatic response through which subjective and group identity are upheld by the act of rejecting anything that threatens a person's body. Kristeva (1982) describes how it is not the "lack of cleanliness or health that causes *abjection*, but what disturbs identity, systems, and order, what does not respect borders, positions, and rules, the in-between, the ambiguous, the composite" (Kristeva, 1982, p. 4).

While Kristeva is not overly concerned with the socially constructive role of *abjection*, Douglas (1966/2001) identifies how acts of defilement, transgression, and that which crosses social boundaries enables opportunities for people to express and uphold certain values and social behaviours as being pure, hygienic, unpolluted, and holy. The act of rejection sets codes of conduct by calling out that which is considered dirty, polluted, or dangerous. This is achieved by responding to transgressive acts by imposing sanctions, punishment, rejection, and public rituals endorsing positive behaviours.

This book will consider how actions of disgust, that which crosses social boundaries and is out of place, is responded to by different members of the prison system. It will explore how these acts are used to police social borders, accrue benefits, as well as perpetuate violence within the prison and contiguous health and social welfare systems. For those involved in the prison system, this forms a society on the margins in which behaviours of violence and disgust, "matter out of place", is used and understood differently from mainstream society.

2.4 Research Methods

2.4.1 Data Collection and Study Sample

This book is the product of an ethnographic study exploring the "lived experience" of 34 men and women living with HIV as they move through a state jail-prison system and return to the community. Participants living with HIV had access to specialised HIV and primary care, mental health services, dental care, and addiction treatment in prison. As inmates returned to the community, they received case management support before their release, during their transition, and for a period after settling in the community. Participants residing in the community also received access to a range of public assistance programmes (e.g., Section 8 Housing and Supplemental Nutrition Assistance Program (SNAP)).

Data was collected between 2011 and 2013. This included 77 semi-structured interviews and participant observations conducted across seven male and female penal facilities (ranging from minimum to super-maximum security) and community-based organisations, including case management support offices, hospitals, and shelters (Appendix A: Study Design; Appendix B: Research Field;). Participants (N = 72), included: short—and long-term inmates in jail/prison (n = 26); prison health-care providers (n = 14); correctional officers and administrators (n = 17); former inmates and family of inmates (n = 9), and physicians and social workers (n = 6). Additional information on the attributes of research participants can be found in Appendix C: Participant Attributes.

Interviews were audio-recorded and conducted in private, confidential settings.

Purposive sampling was used to select a range of institutions, people, and spaces that commonly framed HIV-positive individuals' experiences before, during, and after incarceration and comprise the research setting. Incarcerated HIV-positive participants were identified through an HIV care specialist during a twice-weekly HIV clinic and sampled to include a diversity of inmates based on length of sentence, gender, and prison security classification. These participants were followed up in the community six months after an initial interview. Theoretical and opportunistic sampling techniques were used to recruit prison staff and administrators from a range of facilities (Appendix D: Sampling and Recruitment).

In the community, formerly incarcerated persons living with HIV were recruited through case management services to include a range across gender, length of time living in the community (>12 months), and classification level at last imprisonment. Formerly incarcerated participants were invited to bring family members to community-based interviews. Community health care providers and transitional support staff were purposively recruited through case management services and community HIV services providing care to formerly incarcerated persons. I sought to capture all primary healthcare personnel who treated formerly incarcerated persons with HIV.

Throughout the course of fieldwork, I was allowed to move freely around most Melville prison and jail facilities. Activities with inmates included observation of 250 clinical consultations, sharing meals, public health education, weekly exercise classes, playing card games and socialising, observing intake processing, discharge planning for HIV case management services, and attending 29 parole hearings. Upon inmates' re-entry to the community, fieldwork included observing consultations with case management workers, meetings with shelters, addiction treatment centres, welfare offices, hospice care, and conducting regular home visits.

2.4.2 Data Analysis

Data was analysed using constructivist grounded theory (Charmaz, 2006). Analysis commenced in the field, and observations, rapport building, and the creation of fieldnotes informed subsequent interviews. Hand-written journals of HIV clinical observations, informal conversations, daily routines, and notes detailing observations of relationships, descriptions of physical space, language, and institutional rules, and data from "self-reflection" interviews helped establish emerging ideas and themes.

After completing fieldwork, "line-by-line coding" (Charmaz, 2006, p. 55) was conducted using NVivo 9 software (NVivo, 2010), followed by axial coding to facilitate a process of "following the thread" (i.e., themes, relationships, accounts) throughout the data (Moran-Ellis et al., 2006) and to integrate ethnographic participant observations with interview transcripts from multiple participant subgroups (Appendix E: Empirical Data and Analysis).

2.4.3 Approval and Permissions

Ethical approval for this study was obtained from the London School of Hygiene & Tropical Medicine (Ref. 6052). Study materials were then reviewed and approved by the "Melville" Hospital Institutional Review Board (CMTT/PROJ Ref. 215911). An application and formal presentation were made to, and approval was granted by, the Melville Prison System Medical Research Advisory Group. Informed consent was obtained from each interview participant, and participants were reminded of the researcher's status as an ethnographic researcher during informal conversations, for example, by being explicit about creating field note entries. Pseudonyms were used for institution and participant names to maintain participant confidentiality.

2.5 Immersion into Violence

2.5.1 Experiencing Violence

When doing research for this book, I witnessed the objectification and dehumanisation of inmates, self-harming behaviour, and the physical and social effects of extreme poverty. I observed staff members' frustration, desperation, anger, shame, and fear. Participants revealed painful stories of rape, abuse, suicide attempts, addiction, overdose, stigmatisation, and death. In the community, this witnessing continued as participants returned to their lives on the street and struggled to access resources needed to survive. I often wondered if anyone ever overcomes such challenging life circumstances. As I meditated on this thought, I found myself becoming increasingly angry, depressed, and felt helpless.

There is an allure to witnessing violence when carrying out research on violence, produced by the engagement in violence inherent in ethnographic approaches. Witnessing violence is the method through which it is documented as well as lived. Capturing instances of violence through fieldwork and writing an ethnographic text, including the extreme as well as the mundane, are of interest in the production of a close account of this phenomenon. However, studying violence, especially through ethnographic immersion in a context in which violence is produced, raises real concerns related to not only how an account of violence is represented, but also how the researcher might experience it. The effects of witnessing violence, and the sense of unavoidable complicity, given its structural relations, may be immediately difficult to comprehend, but nevertheless can be personally impactful.

Some of the personal effects of witnessing violence are not always foreseen or predicted and may take shape over time and often in an unpredictable way. The impact of witnessing violence is in the making, and further becomes apparent through reflection in the "re-living" of witnessed events during analysis and the construction of a representative text. This can make responding pragmatically to the personal and emotional effects of conducting difficult fieldwork a challenging task. I was drawn into the violence of this setting through opportunities to witness it, as much as I reacted in relation to, and against, it. The title of Chapter 3 is suggestive of this difficult relationship. "Why would an inmate swallow razor blades?" is an extreme example of much more routine, less visible, less horrific instances of violence both witnessed and experienced. Being drawn into observing extreme violence is an engagement, an embodiment through the affective impacts of the witnessing, with personal consequences that may not be immediately realised or even imagined.

As I reflect on fieldwork and the re-living of what I witnessed through my engagement with data and its write-up, I can see that I became more withdrawn from my daily activities. I found the mental labour of assimilating and accommodating traumatic experiences into my understanding of the world even more challenging than witnessing it, as I was now tasked with having to "really think" about my participants' distress. I was terrified by the task of representing what I was beginning to understand about participants' lives.

Perhaps the embodied effects of witnessed violence in ethnographic fieldwork may become more personally meaningful and consuming, even haunting, after salient events have passed, for the experience of violence does not "pass" and cannot be left behind. In cases of violence structured by its institutional setting, as in my experience in the prison, a sense of complicity in its production through witnessing it meant that others' violence became internalised as a sense of self-deficit, guilt, and sadness. This then, is the process of structural violence in action, a shared sense of violation and complicity in the production of a type of violence experienced by both the researcher and the population being studied.

2.5.2 Writing About Violence

In this book, I take care to describe how new analytical concepts emerged through research participants' language and experiences, drawing links to the systems, politics, and practices integral to their production. Multiple participant accounts across institutions allow for a powerful understanding of how violence is practiced and understood in prison. While violence can be understood as being productive, it does not mean that it is morally good. Exploring and theorising the nuanced ways in which violence can lead to the preservation of people creates new ways of understanding the effects of violence, systems for classifying it, and recognises the spaces where violence takes place.

There is an inherent degree of violence produced when writing about violence. The language used to describe its effects, selection of participant accounts, and setting boundaries for where it can exist is infused in power relationships. Violence can be particularly seductive, and ethnographers must take care not to sensationalise nor sanitise it in their engagement in the field, or when writing about it (Bourgois, 2001). Participants in this study experienced a vulnerability brought about by poverty, structural inequalities, imprisonment, and failing medical and welfare systems. However, it is vital to acknowledge, give voice, and authenticate these individuals' experiences, which are all too often underrepresented in scholarly work.

References

Bourgois, P. (2001). The power of violence in war and peace. *Ethnography, 2*(1), 5–34.

Braman, D. (2007). *Doing time on the outside: Incarceration and family life in Urban America*. Ann Arbor, MI: University of Michigan Press.

Carroll, L. (1974). *Hacks, Blacks, and cons: Race relations in a maximum security prison*. Lanham, MD: Lexington Books.

Charmaz, K. (2006). *Constructing grounded theory: A practical guide through qualitative analysis*. London, UK: Sage Publications.

Clear, T. R. (2007). *Imprisoning communities: How mass incarceration makes disadvantaged neighborhoods worse*. Oxford and New York: Oxford University Press.

Clear, T., Rose, D. R., & Ryder, J. A. (2001). Incarceration and the community: The problem of removing and returning offenders. *Crime & Delinquency, 47*(3), 335–351.

Clemmer, D. (1940). *The prison community*. New York, NY: Rinehart and Winston.

Colaguori, C. (2010). Symbolic violence and violation of human rights: Continuing the sociological critique of domination. *International Journal of Criminology and Sociological Theory, 3*(2), 388–400.

Colvin, M. (1992). *The penitentiary in crisis: Accommodation to riot in New Mexico*. New York, NY: State University of New York Press.

Comfort, M. (2008). *Doing time together: Love and family in the shadow of the Prison*. Chicago, IL: Chicago University Press.

Crouch, B. M. (1980). *The keepers: Prison guards and contemporary corrections*. Springfield, IL: Charles C Thomas Publisher.

Cunha, M. (2014). The ethnography of prisons and penal confinement. *The Annual Review of Anthropology, 43*, 217–233.

Das, V. (1996). The spatialization of violence: Case study of a 'communal riot'. In K. Basu & S. Subrahmanyam (Eds.), *Unravelling the nation: Sectarian conflict and India's secular identity*. New Delhi: Penguin.

Das, V. (2000). The act of witnessing, violence, poisonous knowledge, and subjectivity. In V. Das, A. Kleinman, M. Ramphele, & P. Reynolds (Eds.), *Violence and subjectivity* (pp. 205–225). Berkeley: University of California Press.

Diaz-Cotto, J. (1996). Gender, ethnicity and the state: Latina and Latino prison politics. In S. Easton (Ed.), *Prisoners' rights: Principles and pratice*. New York, NY: State University New York Press.

Douglas, M. (1966/2001). *Purity and danger: An analysis of the concepts of pollution and taboo*. London, UK: Routledge.

Edgar, K., O'Donnell, I., & Martin, C. (2003). *Prison violence: The dynamics of conflict, fear and power*. New York, NY: Routledge.

Esposito, M. (2012). "Double burden": A qualitative study of HIV positive prisoners in Italy. *International Journal of Prison Health, 8*(1), 35–44.

Fleisher, M. S. (1989). *Warehousing violence*. Newbury Park, CA: Sage.

Haley, D. F., Golin, C. E., Farel, C. E., Wohl, D. A., Scheyett, A. M., Garrett, J. J., … Parker, S. (2014). Multilevel challenges to engagement in HIV care after prison release: a theory-informed qualitative study comparing prisoners' perspectives before and after community reentry. *BMC Public Health, 14*, 1–15.

Hann, W. (2008). Violence as an essentially contested concept. In S. Body-Gendrot & P. Spierendburg (Eds.), *Violence in Europe* (pp. 27–40). New York, NY: Springer.

Irwin, J. (1970). *The felon*. Englewood Cliffs, NJ: Prentice-Hall.

Irwin, J. (1980). *Prisons in turmoil*. Boston, MA: Little, Brown.

Irwin, J. (1985). *The jail: Managing the underclass in American society*. Berkeley, CA: University of California Press.
Irwin, J., & Cressey, D. (1962). Thieves, convicts and the inmate culture. *Social Problems, 10,* 142–155.
Jacobs, J. (1977). *Stateville: The penitentiary in mass society Chicago,* IL: University of Chicago Press.
Jauregui, B. (2013). Dirty anthropology: Epistemologies of violence and ethical entanglements in police ethnography. In W. Garriott (Ed.), *Policing and contemporary governance: The anthropology of police in pratice*. New York, NY: Palgrave Macmillan.
Kleinman, A. (2000). The violence of everday life: The multiple forms and dynamics of social violence. In V. Das, A. Kleinman, M. Ramphele, & P. Reynolds (Eds.), *Violence and subjectivity* (pp. 226–241). Berkeley, CA: University of California Press.
Kristeva, J. (1982). *Powers of horror: An essay on abjection* (L. S. Roudiez, Trans.). New York, NY: Columbia University Press.
Kruttschnitt, C., & Gartner, R. (2005). *Marking time in the Golden State: women's imprisonment in California*. Cambridge, UK and New York: Cambridge University Press.
Marquart, J. W. (1986). Doing research in prisons: The strength and weakness of full participation as a guard. *Justice Quarterly, 3*(1), 15–32.
McCorkel, A. J. (2003). Embodied surveillance and the gendering of punishment. *Journal of Contemporary Ethnography, 31*(1), 41–76.
Moran-Ellis, J., Alexander, V. D., Cronin, A., Dickinson, M., Fielding, J., Sleney, J., & Thomas, H. (2006). Triangulation and integration: Processes, claims and implications. *Qualitative Research, 6*(1), 45–59.
Nunn, A., Cornwall, A., Fu, J., Bazerman, L., Loewenthal, H., & Bekwith, C. (2010). Linking HIV-positive jail inmates to treatment, care, and social services after release: Results from a qualitative assessment of the COMPASS program. *Journal of Urban Health, 87,* 954–968.
Nvivo. (2010). NVivo qualitative data analysis software (Version 9): QSR International Pty Ltd.
Owen, B. (1998). *In the mix: Struggle and survival in a women's prison.* Albany, NY: State University of New York Press.
Philliber, S. (1987). Thy brothers keeper: A review of the literature on correctional officers. *Justice Quarterly, 4*(1), 9–37.
Rhodes, L. A. (2001). Toward an anthropology of prisons. *Annual Review of Anthropology, 30,* 65–83.

Rhodes, L. A. (2004). *Total confinement: Madness and reason in the maximum security prison.* Berkeley, CA: University of California Press.

Small, W., Wood, E., Betteridge, G., Montaner, J., & Kerr, T. (2009). The impact of incarceration upon adherence to HIV treatment among HIV-positive injection drug users: A qualitative study. *AIDS Care, 21*(6), 708–714.

Sykes, G. M. (1958). *The society of captives: A study of maximum security prison.* Princeton, NJ: Princeton University Press.

Trammell, R. (2012). *Enforcing the convict code: Violence and prison culture.* Boulder, CO: Lynne Rienner.

Wacquant, L. (2002). The curious eclipse of prison ethnography in the age of mass incarceration. *Ethnography, 3*(4), 371–397.

Wacquant, L. (2013). *Deadly symbiosis: Race and the rise of the penal state.* Cambridge, UK: Polity.

Ward, D., & Kassebaum, G. G. (1965). *Women's prison: Sex and social structure.* Piscataway, NJ: Transaction Publishers.

Wilkinson, I. (2013). The problem of suffering as a driving force of rationalization and social change. *The British Journal of Sociology, 64*(1).

Zimmer, L. E. (1986). *Women guarding men.* Chicago, IL: Chicago University Press.

3

Why Would An Inmate Swallow Razor Blades?

Nina, a nurse in Women's Maximum, introduced me to the notion of degradation by recounting an inmate who swallowed razor blades. On my way to interview Nina, I lit a cigarette and walked across the prison yard. Arriving at Women's Maximum, I showed the duty officer my badge, walked up a staircase, and entered a second-floor counselling room. The room was minimally furnished, with a simple metal desk and two plastic chairs. Typically, you could hear women yelling above the noise of the dayroom television, competing with the blare of The Jerry Springer Show. However, the block was quiet on this day, as inmates were confined to their rooms during a routine lockdown. This provided time to interview a member of staff.

I met with Nina several times before conducting a formal interview. She worked in the women's medical dispensary, where I met participants and observed HIV clinics. At the time of this study, Nina was in her seventh year of correctional nursing. While she mostly cared for female offenders, it was not uncommon for her to pick up shifts in other facilities. Nina arrived at the interview in a loose-fitting pink and turquoise uniform. A bob haircut and thick-rimmed glasses sharply framed her round face.

L. Kuester, *Violence in Pursuit of Health*, Palgrave Studies in Prisons and Penology, https://doi.org/10.1007/978-3-030-61350-1_3

During the interview, I asked Nina to illustrate a typical challenge in her daily role as a nurse. She described an inmate who swallowed razor blades in protest for what he believed to be insufficient medical care. Nina explained, "this guy wanted attention; they are always seeking attention". The self-harming inmate had reported himself to an officer, who escorted him to the medical dispensary, where Nina performed a clinical assessment. The inmate was then sent to a local hospital where he received a surgical consultation. Nina claimed that it "was then, and only then, he would be taken away from the prison care that he was objecting".

After surgery, the inmate received a psychological evaluation for his behaviour. Nina described that when the inmate returned to prison, he threatened prison staff with litigation because he was denied a razor blade, an object permitted to him for personal hygiene. She explained, "I have mixed feelings when someone eats a hundred razor blades, we save them, and then we give him back his razor after six-months because he has the right to have it. Does that make sense to you? I don't think that asshole should ever have them again".

First and foremost, it is important to recognise the extreme danger placed on the inmate who self-harmed in Nina's account. His actions can lead to extreme bodily damage or death. The inmate's behaviour would likely carry other sanctions, including segregation or loss of "good time"; a sentence reduction given to prisoners maintaining good behaviour in prison. There is also a loss of dignity he experienced by destroying his body in order to receive rights and resources, including medical attention.

Nina's story illustrates how inmates engage in destructive behaviour to activate a legal protocol, which, in turn, opened a claims-making process for resources otherwise not accessible to them. The inmate's behaviour enabled access to alternative healthcare. The psychological evaluation he received created medical documentation, which could be used to make appeals for welfare support in the future. Having a disability status made it easier for him to access several prisoner re-entry programmes. The threat of a lawsuit, whether successful or not, also provided this inmate with a sense of agency through the potential of financial remuneration.

These actions, in the context of imprisonment, can lead to change in immediate circumstances, and secure resources for an imagined future.

While not explicit in Nina's story, the inmate, Nina, and the officer were aware of why the inmate engaged in destructive behaviour. An inmate's destructive actions and how staff respond and manage this behaviour are part of a quintessential and well-rehearsed social process referred to by some members of the prison as "prison games".

"Degradation" and "prison games" are central themes described in this book. Therefore, it is important to be clear about what these terms mean in the context of imprisonment:

Degradation

Degradation refers to *abjectionable*, illicit, or un-citizenly behaviour done for the pursuit of rights and resources. This chapter introduces three forms of degradation in relation to healthcare delivery: self-degradation, degradation done by others, and structural degradation. Degradation happens in settings where choice is restricted. This condition can lead to a person's empowerment through a claims-making process, while at the same time propelling them into a state of violence and ruination.

Prison Games

Prison games comprise the relational-social process whereby degradation is performed. Inmates and staff used degradation to pursue resources, manage disruptive behaviour, and uphold social and moral boundaries. "Game playing" implies that things are fluid, up for negotiation, and involve the use of social and physical tactics. The idea of a game suggests that there are explicit and implicit rules around how people should act, but these rules are open to disruption and negotiation, around which inmates and staff can navigate and play to their advantages or others' disadvantages.

Not everyone experienced the effects of degradation in the same way. A person's perception of degradation depends on their understanding of the regularity of this social practice, what is at risk during game playing, how agency is gained in other contexts of their lives, and whether or not individuals were able to recognise the accrued effects of degradation over time. Thus, some practices of game playing are, in fact, harmless or free of degradation effect.

3.1 Accessing Healthcare

At the time of this study, Melville prison offered medical and mental health, dental, and health education services. All offenders were eligible for services, including those sentenced and awaiting trial. "Sick calls" and certain clinics operated in all facilities, while infirmary care was only available in select institutions. An on-call practitioner was always available to inmates.

Specialty medical services included HIV care, cardiology, and orthopedic care. Acute medical and surgical interventions were delivered through a partnership with community hospitals, accessed by inmates through "medical furloughs". The prison also hosted medical students and residents. On-site clerks oversaw healthcare billing and electronic record-keeping.

Melville's nursing programme comprised a General Director of Nursing, several nursing supervisors, and 43 licensed nurses. Nursing staff rotated through all prison facilities 24 hours a day, seven days a week. The prison employed several nurse practitioners and clinical nurse specialists.

Inmates first encounter medical services as part of their intake health assessment, typically conducted by a nurse. Nurses also determine inmates' daily access to services through a paper request system. If an inmate wanted to see a healthcare provider, they were required to "put in a slip" to an officer.

The management of medical slips was critical to the co-production of degradation and the playing of prison games. The slip system affects all inmates, not just those living with HIV. A desk nurse was responsible for the daily review of inmates' medical request slips and determining if further medical attention was warranted, effectively acting as a gatekeeper to other healthcare providers in the prison.

I observed several nurses reviewing slips to determine who could access care and on what grounds. Slips were used by nursing staff to render punishment, "settle scores", and police inmates' behaviour by upholding certain morals, as *they* decided who was deserving of attention.

Dotty, a nurse in Men's Jail, exemplified the process of reviewing medical slips. Reading a slip aloud, she said, "I've got bad pain from my hernia" the slips will tell me you know, if they're really, really drug-seeking. "I look up what they are in for [...] and if he's coming up with 'I have a hernia', or 'I have this', and he hasn't reported any of this, and he's in for drugs, get away". She proceeded to toss the slip into a bin before moving on to the next request. Dotty explained that her rejection of the slip was about protecting state resources, as well as upholding the notion that inmates deserve pain: "You see, they just want the State to pay for them. The ones that come in with a hernia, that it's always excruciating pain, and it's reducible and it's like this size [indicating], no, we're not going to do anything for you, and then they [inmates] get pissed off".

Dotty was one of several staff members who viewed requests in this way. For example, Gina, also a nurse in Men's Jail, regularly demonstrated her mistrust for the inmate's requesting care. She explained, "Many of them [inmates] want attention. And it's amazing, you're out there on the streets for eight years at a time, and as soon as you get in front of me, suddenly you have tooth pain that's unbearable. No dude, I think it's bullshit. Most of them are bullshit".

Nurses' refusal to engage with medical requests meant that some inmates went without care or, as illustrated in this chapter, caused them to progressively degrade their bodies in such a way that care could no longer be ignored. In her own words, Dotty explained how degrading behaviours would escalate over time as inmates continued to seek care, "the slips become more creative as inmates discuss with one another what to write".

Nursing staff regularly enforced moral principles by rejecting slips, knowing its consequences on the inmate's health. I spoke with Angel, an inmate in Men's Minimum, after his HIV progressed to AIDS, eventually drawing the attention of a specialist HIV doctor. Angel had developed a fever and ulcers across his body, a clear presentation of illness. I had also talked with the dispensary desk nurse to figure out what happened.

Angel boycotted his medication, feeling he needed to choose between treatment or experience stigmatisation from his fellow inmates. Attending the HIV clinic was concerning because it meant others would know his status. He made multiple requests that his medication be "kept on person" (KOP), but these were all denied by the nurse. For a low-risk offender in Men's Minimum, KOP would normally be allowed. However, Angel claimed his request slips had been rejected because "They [nurses] don't understand, I don't do English perfect". The process made him feel "angry and stupid".

The attending nurse, who was a first-generation American, told me why he withheld care to Angel. Explaining, "he [Angel] should learn English, my parents came to this country and they learned English, and they work a job". This nurse's response is telling for what it reveals; at least for some healthcare providers, inmates were seen to be undeserving and not full members of society. It places health services, what should be a site of care, as a site for punishment.

3.2 Self-degradation

The rejection of slips, while causing delayed care to those in need, also encouraged inmates' response. Dotty mentioned that slips become more creative over time. However, what happens when creative writing fails? Inmates responded to the denial of treatment in different ways, but typically their response involved a degree of "self-degradation", harm to their body in order to achieve the desired outcome of healthcare.

It was January and snowing. I warmed my hands on the only working heater in my Jeep, which was parked in the lot at Women's Maximum. It must have been noon, as the women formed a line along the perimeter, flanked by officers. They would be finishing "chow" at this time, collecting their commissary, and returning to the dorms. Dressed in tan coats, the women fidgeted to keep warm while officers took the count.

Judy, an inmate, waved me over. As I approached, she lowered the paper towels she held over her mouth. She was missing teeth and her gums were bleeding. She explained, "I got twelve of them out today, Landon. Almost all gone".

Years of smoking crack had taken its toll on Judy's dental hygiene. She had been petitioning the prison to get them fixed, and on that day the dentist removed 12 of her upper teeth. However, Judy expressed her concern, as her time in Melville was ending and she was worried that her dentures would not be ready upon her departure, explaining, "They just don't want to pay for it. It is unfair, how am I supposed to eat now? I must do something; I cannot leave here like this".

Judy's situation was not uncommon. Delays in care, particularly for short-term inmates returning to communities with limited or no healthcare, became urgent. Nina explained how inmates like Judy might resolve their situation by using both their bodies and the prison's expected infraction system. She explained, "I've known girls who have stated that they will stay in trouble until their dentures are complete because they're not going to go home without teeth. So, they'll just incite a fight, stay three more months in segregation, see the dentist and get them."

3.2.1 Faking Symptoms

When submitting slips was unsuccessful and generating more prison time was not an option, some inmates faked illness symptoms to gain access to care. On one hand, this action lowered an inmate's dignity, placing them in a position where they feel the need to lie or embellish illness. On the other hand, it perpetuated what many nurses already believe, that inmates are faking it. Caught up in this act of degradation are inmates with medical needs not being met by the healthcare system. Gina, a nurse in Men's Jail, described catching an inmate in this act:

> The kid comes through the hallway, and I can see him. He starts moonwalking, doing Michael Jackson, and pushing himself from wall to wall. He is doing everything. Jumping jacks to increase his heart rate. And so, I just walked outside of the dispensary, and I am standing in the hallway with a "Is that so?" look on my face. And lo and behold he comes around the corner and grabs his chest, oh, he is having a hard time [...] So I said, "Well, what was that all about?" And he says, "What? I just threw up in my cell". I said, "Young man, we've got cameras all over this facility. I just watched you imitate Michael Jackson, jumping jacks, the whole nine yards".

I had frequently observed similar accounts to what Gina described, wondering if what I was witnessing was genuine or a performance. For example, Big Jay, an inmate in Men's Medium, met with an HIV specialist during a clinical rotation. He winced with every movement, barely able to erect himself from his wheelchair and onto the examination table. I was struck by how he relentlessly lobbied the physician to increase his pain meds and a bottom bunk or private cell. He also asked for growth hormones and nutrition drinks, careful to provide a rationale for each of his requests. As Big Jay left the clinic, a nurse took me aside and said: "you know he is faking it, right?".

Later that day, I too had shared in the nurse's suspicion. Walking through the prison yard, I watched as Big Jay jogged the perimeter. We clocked eyes. Big Jay had immediately returned to, what I suspect to be, a performance of illness. He stopped in his tracks, limped, and clutched the wall for support.

3.2.2 Evidence of a Damaged Body

Bodily harm was the swiftest way for inmates to receive medical attention, as it provided indisputable evidence of a medical need. However, the harm would need to be exceptionally severe and life-threatening. Pep, a retired officer, described how self-harming behaviour was common in prison, saying: "I think in my six years or seven years as an officer I've had 14 attempted suicides. People cutting themselves. Hanging seems to have sort of taken off a little bit more now."

Inmates used their viral load, blood, urine, and faeces to gain access to care. Sometimes inmate's self-harming acts would garner medical attention, other times not. Often self-inflicted damage worsened over time, as inmates pushed their bodies towards total destruction.

The dispensary radio chirped, "code blue, code blue". I could hear Officer Atwood yelling at an inmate, "you want to behave, you fucking piece of shit, you're not going to win with us". Their exchange became muted over the sound of slamming doors, the holler of inmates, coughing, chains, boots on the floor, and the continued chirp of the radio.

Curious, I had peered from the dispensary door and saw six officers escorting a bleeding inmate towards me. I felt a sting in my throat and coughed uncontrollably. Noticing my struggle, a nurse handed me a mask, saying, "here kid, take one of these. Don't worry, you will get used to it". A cloud of pepper spray had filled the dispensary as the men approached.

The inmate replied to Officer Atwood; "fuck you, go fuck yourself". Snot and blood dripped from the inmate's face and stained the collar of his uniform. He screamed out "my eyes, my eyes, my fucking eyes, please just wipe my eyes". Another responding officer replied, "are you going to behave?" This enraged the inmate, who shouted: "I'm going to keep doing this, I'm going to keep smashing my head, I don't give a fuck".

Officers brought this inmate to the dispensary for a medical assessment. He was placed under the shower to wash the chemicals from his eyes. The officers walked the inmate to a psychiatric observation cell and stripped him naked at the door. He was cuffed to the bed, first his ankles then his wrists. The inmate continued to scream, now jerking his arms so that the metal cuffs would break his skin. A nurse provided a rapid assessment of his head, tossed a blanket over his genitals, and, along with the officers, left the cell.

The inmate received medical attention. He was also removed from the general offender population and placed into a private observation cell. He was disciplined for hitting his head against a bedpost, for which his motivation was unknown.

3.3 Degradation by Others

"Degradation by others", or active degradation, is an example that goes beyond the situationally produced self-harming behaviour of inmates in order to consider harmful acts or abdications by staff who withheld care to create punishment. These acts, and the process through which they are produced, were done in response to inmates' self-degradation, and sometimes used to police moral boundaries in relation to who is deserving of care.

3.3.1 Delayed or Denied Care

Resentments turned into actions, as nurses sought to "set things straight" by rendering healthcare as a site of punishment. Linda, a nurse in Women's Maximum, voiced her anger towards inmates who she believed used prison as an opportunity to access specific resources. Linda thought welfare assistance should only be reserved for certain members of the public, not offenders, she explained:

> I very rarely get somebody say, "I'm on Blue Cross, Blue Shield", or very rarely, it's either they have no insurance whatsoever, or "Oh, well, I have pending SSI. They're pending. I'm trying to get on SSI for this disability". Let me just throw this out to you. My grandfather had polio his whole life, he was in a wheelchair, crutches, wheelchair, crutches, and supported a wife and eight kids. Never bitched, never received one red cent of state funds. Do you know what? The only disability you have is none. You do not have a disability, you're a con artist. Now get out of my face.

Other nurses rendered healthcare as a site of degradation through delaying treatment. Gina, in Men's Jail, did this when she "slow-walked" a medication refill for an offender convicted of assaulting a minor. Gina recounted her interaction with this inmate, saying, "Oh, you have a problem sleeping? Oh, did you rape those children? Well, I will give you 300 milligrammes of Trazodone. Hey, if it doesn't work, just put in the slip, I'll increase it to 4'. Do you see what I am saying? Like are you serious? Do you know what? Suffer, you son of a bitch".

John, a nurse in Men's Minimum, described a colleague who withheld drug detox protocols to offenders. He recounted his conversation with an inmate who suffered because of his colleague's action:

> He [inmate] says "John, man, listen, I've been sick. I came in. I shot heroin up". And I'll say, "I'll put you on a CIWA [*Clinical Institute Withdrawal Assessment]* protocol". And then the nurse will say, "You saw so-and-so today?" I said "Yeah". "I told him to put a slip in". "Well, he's actively withdrawing. We have the medication right in this closet to help him out. Why are you going to make the guy wait? Oh, because your ex-husband was a drug addict". I know, you know, this provider in here

that her husband was a drug addict, and she hates drug addicts, so she makes them suffer.

3.3.2 Requiring Performances

Degradation by others happened when nursing staff required performances of sickness in order to justify care. Nurses used the threat of infractions and moments of humiliation to withhold care. For example, Janjak, a nurse in Men's Minimum, described "testing" inmates to determine if an illness was genuine or rehearsed:

Janjak: Some will come to me and say, "I've been having diarrhoea the whole night". I say, "How many times have you had bowel movements?" They say, "20 times". I say, "like how often?" They say, "like every five minutes". I say, "you've been having diarrhoea every five minutes starting when?" They say, "starting at 12:30"... "wow, we've been talking here for 30 minutes, so you don't have diarrhoea".

Landon: What do they say to that?

Janjak: They say, they do not know, it just stopped. You know when somebody has diarrhoea. The thing will be as calm as mine. And then you say "okay, take this cup. Go to that bathroom. Bring me a cupful of faeces". "Oh, no, I don't think I'll be able to do that".

[...]

Janjak: They want to stay out of work. So, we say, "If I give you this slip to stay out of work, you do not have your visit [visitation]" and they say "Oh, I'll go to work".

Landon: So, you must make it difficult?

Janjak: Yes, exactly. You are going to stretch it a little bit so that the truth will come out. The truth will come out, the truth, because I work with these guys, I know them very well. I always know the truth.

3.3.3 Talking Back

Degradation by others also happened through verbal abuse. Staff were often able to say whatever they liked, while inmates were punished for "talking back". Chaney, an inmate in Men's Jail, described this behaviour at *med line*, the process, and place where medications were delivered to inmates, explaining:

> Nurses say like "Move back to the fucking line", and "Get your hands out of your fucking pants". I mean, the way they talk. They are not talking to me like that, because I would say something, and then I would have gone to segregation, booked or in seg.

Inmate's use of foul language often resulted in segregation. Staff also used this language to elicit a comparable response from inmates, which also resulted in segregation. Cam, and inmate in Men's Jail, described how segregation was a more restrictive site for care:

> They will come by at med line time at night, before they shut the facility down, and they will skip right by your cell. Little devious-ass shit like that. Or the nurse will be in the block, and you will ask for a med slip. They will not give it to you. Petty shit. In the morning time the trap will be open, and instead of the nurse coming down to give you your meds, they will just walk right by your cell.

3.4 Structural Degradation

3.4.1 The Legal Foundation for Care

The introduction to this book outlines the demographic, political, and legal conditions that frame the delivery of healthcare in prison. I also describe how healthcare in the community, for those involved in the criminal justice system, can be challenging to obtain upon re-entry. Prison is the only space where medical care is constitutionally mandated ("Estelle v. Gamble, 429 U.S. 97," 1976), positioning it as an essential site for public health delivery.

The Estelle v. Gamble ruling entitles inmates to professional medical judgement, diagnoses, and access to treatment. Any disallowance of medical care must meet standards of "deliberate indifference" to "serious medical needs" in order to run afoul of the Eighth Amendment of the

U.S. Constitution. However, as mentioned earlier, ruling's wording is particularly problematic for the delivery of routine care in prison by enabling negligible care.

This ruling's language has led to several legal case studies demonstrating staff delaying care to inmates, and are reluctant to test, diagnose, or seek outside consultation (Thompson, 2010). Thompson describes, what can be observed through degradation practices, that staff withhold care from inmates out of feeling manipulated (Thompson, 2010, p. 636). Further, legal studies show that allegations of manipulation are most frequently levelled against inmates who are most steadfast in their pursuit of treatment, "making their illness so obvious that they cannot be accused of lying" (Thompson, 2010, p. 648).

3.4.2 No Medical Grievance, No Justice

The correctional handbook states, "consistent with [Melville] policy governing inmate grievance procedures, medical decisions are not grievable". Thus, there was no formal mechanism for inmates to file a medical-related complaint. Inmates could not select who delivered their care, nor the treatments prescribed. This meant that inmates faced restricted choices when experiencing potential maltreatment.

Instead, inmates were encouraged to write letters to the prison healthcare administrator. While this is not a grievance, it would register their concern. At the time of this study, according to the deputy director, there were over 900 letters of complaint from inmates and their families during a 12-month period. The deputy director explained how complaints were reviewed, "my assistant goes in the medical record, and goes to the date, checks the issue, sees if it's true. Sees if the guy was seen, if the medication was ordered, and if it wasn't ordered". This explanation provided little insight into the process of resolving complaints and, what, if any, actions were taken to prevent future offenses.

John, a nurse in Men's Minimum, clarified that administrators occasionally followed up on letters of concern. However, he believed that complaints were not always addressed, most inmates did not know whom to contact about their concerns, and many feared reprisals for complaining. John said, "I'm always telling [Tommy, his nursing supervisor] there should be some kind of a sign in a well-lit area where the inmates can say 'If I have a problem, I can write this person', and feel confident that it's going to get there, and there's going to be no repercussions".

Numerous legal barriers prevented inmates from undertaking litigation of medical misconduct. While the Federal Tort Claims Act grants inmates the right to sue for medical negligence, the Eleventh Amendment of the U.S. Constitution prohibits federal courts from entertaining claims against the State (Wool, 2007, pp. 30–31). Consequently, inmates can only sue individual government staff members. However, many government staff have qualified immunity against civil lawsuits, which can include nurses and officers.

The Litigation Reform Act (PLRA) can put up additional barriers for inmates to litigate complaints (Wool, 2007). PLRA restricts inmates from filing successive petitions for a grievance to be tried in The Court. It also requires all filers to pay a $350–450 filing fee. The PLRA places restrictions on attorney's fees, requiring unsuccessful inmates to incur all deposition costs, restrictions that deter poor inmates from filing, as well as legal representation from taking up cases. PLRA also mandates an "exhaustion rule", which requires inmates to use all internal grievance procedures before filing a lawsuit, and that this process follows an administrative timeline of two to four weeks (Boston, 2006). There are additional restrictions on the types of cases The Court will hear. For example, if your grievance is for mental and emotional distress, The Court is restricted from prosecuting a prisoner's injury in the absence of substantial physical damage (Boston, 2006).

3.4.3 Punishment Regime

The prison was also a space that embraced a punishment regime. In this setting, infractions, even minor ones, had the predictable consequence of solitary confinement, loss of meritorious good time, and protocols for psychological evaluation or placement on suicide watch. These institutional procedures, while on the one hand served to deliver punishment, on the other hand, were used by inmates to maneuver themselves within the prison institution and take control of their release date or enable access to certain healthcare provisions.

3.5 No One Is Exempt

The lived experience of degradation and prison games was not something experienced by everyone in the same way. Different Groups of inmates had access to different resources, had agency in other aspects of their lives, and each inmate might internalise moments of degradation differently. However, the nature of degradation is that it is structural, so no one would be exempt from its effects.

3.5.1 HIV-Positive

In this book, people living with HIV provide first-hand accounts of degradation as it is lived. However, HIV-positive inmates might experience degradation differently from other inmates. Their HIV status granted them access to specific resources and relationships, thereby changing the field where games are played.

Aspects of prison healthcare were overseen by HIV specialists operating on the periphery of game playing, including community medical consultants, re-entry specialists, and a public health nurse. HIV-positive inmates leaving prison were eligible to receive case management support, HIV treatment, primary medical care, addiction treatment, mental health, health insurance programmes, and other public assistance.

Keith, an inmate in Men's Jail, had multiple co-morbidities that required him to make regular trips to the medical dispensary. For some inmates, this level of engagement with the slip system resulted in increased game playing, however, Keith had other options, explaining, "Some people, it takes a few weeks. But I never put a slip in, because [HIV specialist] always calls me up to the dispensary".

In the context of re-entry, one's HIV status enabled some assurances to external resources, for which others might need to play games to receive (described in Chapter 4). Romeo, an inmate in Men's Medium, explained, "Well, they helped me. They got my bus passes, my resources, food. Put me in connection with different organisations that I didn't know existed until I got HIV". Conversely, the "special status" of HIV also made inmates a target for game playing in other ways, as a senior administrator explained:

> They [HIV specialists] prescribe things that do not even make sense. Double mattresses, double pillows. HIV is not a very painful disease historically. Why does this guy need two mattresses, you know? Because then, what ends up happening is that group of individuals, because of their diagnosis, become a privileged group.

Linda, a nurse in Women's Maximum, described how staff viewed the care provided by community-based specialists, suggesting how their actions might influence the game:

> I think a lot of the nurses are hostile. I will never forget the day that Dr. Goldman [HIV specialist] brought in doughnuts for the nurses at Intake, and they wouldn't eat them, and they put some like nasty remark on them. It's a hostility. I'll look at them and think, "Why are you doing this [providing care], and why do you encourage this?"

3.5.2 Mentally Ill

Hugo, an inmate in Men's Supermax, was an example of someone living with schizophrenia in prison. He was removed from the general population into segregation because of his disruptive behaviour, which I suspect was an effect of mental illness. He was convicted for sexually assaulting a minor, an offense that brought about additional punishment from staff.

Hugo entered the meeting room, escorted by an officer. He wore shackles on his wrists and ankles. The escorting officer sat in front of a window looking onto the room, a security requirement of the facility. Throughout the interview, the officer rapped on the glass with his knuckles, taunting Hugo by quietly mouthing "child diddler". In response, Hugo sat close to my side in order to reply to my questions with whispers.

He was regularly denied toilet paper by prison staff and told to "shit like a dog". Hugo responded to this officer by acting out, which resulted in additional punishments. I cannot be sure why staff, in this case, an officer, denied Hugo's request for toilet paper. However, I suspect it was done out of punishment for disruptive behaviour, and to uphold moral boundaries given Hugo's offense. Hugo recounted his exchange with an officer:

> One day I have no toilet paper. I wanted to use the bathroom so badly. He [officer] refused to give me the toilet paper. I started to kick the door, and the officer came over and started screaming. He calls me Freddy Kruger, motherfucker, all kinds of shit. They called the lieutenant, and the lieutenant said, "did you take his shoes off?" And he said, "Yeah, I took his shoes off, but he keeps on kicking the door". So, they booked me, they gave me 25 [days] for that.

The mentally ill represent a particularly tragic group of inmates in prison. Facilities were not equipped to provide the necessary support, so many problematic mentally ill inmates would reside in segregation. Hugo's inclusion in prison games demonstrates staff reluctance to allow inmates such as Hugo to move from identities of criminal to ill. Recognising that Hugo was "not in his right mind" would have undermined the punishment role of the prison. I cannot help but wonder to what degree Hugo, and inmates like him, are fully aware of their involvement in prison games.

3.6 "Prison Games" in Healthcare

The research focus on HIV-positive inmates enabled an up-close examination of prison healthcare. A key theme arising from the data suggests that prison games were central to a person's agency under conditions of remarkable constraint. Therefore, it was important to consider the interplay between "structure" and "agency" in everyday practice (Bourdieu, 1977). In Melville Prison, playing games was integral to the prison "structure", as it was replete with pre-given expectations for how someone was expected to behave under institutional rules and laws. In the context of prison, "agency" was often expressed through different forms of degradation. Bourdieu's "theory of practice" offers a formula from which to view the practice of prison games: [(*Habitus*) (Capital) + Field = Practice] (Bourdieu, 1984/2010, p. 95).

Prison games were quintessential to correctional healthcare. Moments of degradation functioned as "capital" by enabling individuals to uphold or change their position within the prison and peri-carceral space. For example, self-degradation enabled an inmate's control over objects, space, and time in the present, as well as access to finance, housing, and other benefits in the future. Degradation done by staff members policed moral and social boundaries of the field by imposing beliefs about *who* is deserving of benefits and care.

3.6.1 The Field of Prison Games

Bourdieu depicts the "field" as a network of configurations and objective relations between different members' positions. The field is defined in members' existence and in the determinations imposed upon other occupants, agents, or institutions, by their present and potential situations and in the structure of the distribution of power. A member's capital commands them access to specific profits at stake in the field, and understood in relation to their objective relations to other members' positions (Bourdieu & Wacquant, 1992, p. 97).

The field of prison games was where staff and inmates negotiated social positions and where capital was accrued and lost. The "rules of the game" were not simply imposed or fixed, but rather actions and ways of being were engendered and, at the same time, limited by structuring mechanisms. Prison games were simultaneously structured and constitutive of the field's future structure (Christoforou & Lainé, 2014, p. 165). There were rules, for example, legal entitlements that determined the quality of medical care, institutional booking procedures for "infractions", and rewards for good behaviour. Playing to these rules enabled members' control over both space and time. Tactics of degradation were learned explicitly and implicitly by different members. To "play the game" was a metaphor that described the continuous struggle between staff and inmates as they attempted to change or safeguard their positions in the field.

3.6.2 Inmate Habitus

A persons position in the field results from the interplay between *habitus*, power afforded to their position, and the accumulation or loss of capital enabling movement within the field (Calhoun, LiPuama, & Postone, 1993, p. 5). *Habitus* can be understood as the "internalisation of externality". It is the imprint of society on a person's lasting disposition through trained capacities and structured propensities to think, feel, and act in a certain way. It guides someone to respond in creative ways to the constraints and solicitations of their external milieu (Wacquant, 2005, p. 316 as cited in Navarro, 2006, p. 16). Therefore, *habitus* is engendered through the interaction between "structure" and "practice" and through on-going, often-thoughtless, processes that become internalised as second nature.

For inmates, *habitus* was engendered through historical and on-going violence in prison and the community. For many, this included social and health depravations depicted in the introduction of this book. To overcome such deprivations, prison games and destructive behaviour was used to secure otherwise unattainable capital. For example, inmates "learned to hustle", a common strategy to make money through entering illicit business on the street. This had the expected consequence of returning to prison over time. The prison was "time away" for inmates, where some freedoms were suspended, and dignity lowered, for the pursuit of capital gains. In this case, capital might include a person's removal from threats in the community, access to drug detoxification, and entry into a routinised structure that enabled time to work on one's health and wellbeing. Prison games were learned collectively and independently. Some inmates gained implicit knowledge through exposure to a shared environment and similar biographical histories, while others learned to play the game through more overt knowledge-sharing.

For less the experienced inmates in prison, game playing was learned through trial-and-error during their interactions with staff. Game playing started with small moments of degradation, such as faking medical symptoms but quickly escalated to grievous bodily harm. The process of being "tested" by inmates was particularly common for new staff members, and no one in the prison was immune from this experience. Reflecting on fieldnotes, it was not unusual for an inmate during an interview to ask for access to a phone or help with benefits paperwork, which over time escalated to include requests for contraband and help to obtain institutional privileges. Pep, a retired officer, explained that this escalation of behaviour was done, in part, to determine if someone "played by the books" (followed the rules), or if they were open to negotiations, explaining:

> You will say there is no harm in that, and, do you know what? There is no harm in me taking that letter and mailing it for them. Obviously, you cannot do it. But do you know what? That is the first thing. That is the start of it. Then it goes on to something else, then something else, till they are finally like "I've got him".

Senior inmates, known as "career criminals", passed down their knowledge to younger inmates, known as "kids". Gina, a nurse in Men's Jail, depicted how healthcare staff perceived career criminals:

> Oh, the guys [career criminals] have been here a long time and are very smart. They know how to get things; they know who to see. As soon as they walk in that door, they say "I didn't have any healthcare, but now I do". And they will walk in, the ones who have been here a long time, "I need glasses, I need dentures. I need my meds".

Some career criminals held specialised cultural knowledge, which afforded them a special status in prison. For example, Rahim, an inmate in Men's Maximum, had legal expertise around playing prison games. Rahim had been in prison for over 15 years at the time of the study.

He was serving two counts of life, consecutive and without parole. He referred to himself as the "jailhouse lawyer" because of his expansive knowledge of the internal grievance procedures and wider juridical-legal system. He explained his role:

> And I told him [prison officer] one day, I says "I'm not here just to do my legal stuff and focus on me. If I can, I help other people" And I have, and I've won a lot of Family Court cases for guys in here.

While career criminals often departed knowledge to kids orally, there was some evidence that information was shared through written material. Garth, a senior health administrator, described this the written material circulated widely within the prison system. He depicted a "how to get on SSI" text that was circulating in prison:

> They have tracked a really accurate book that the inmates created. It gives them instructions on how to get on SSI [welfare benefits]. [...] It tells you absolutely what not to do, and what not to say, and what State not to say it in. Do not say you have mental illness in California, because they track everything there. So, say you had mental illness, and you used to live in Michigan. You ran away from home, your father abused you. And it comes into the same story all the time. [...] "All those records are sealed, no one can get them". You can say whatever you want about when you were a child. You attempted suicide when you were 16 years old, you were molested by your stepfather, your stepfather or whoever, and it is an automatic one-year benefits.

3.6.3 Staff Habitus

Chapters 5 and 6 will describe the milieu of prison staff culture and explore their motivations for playing prison games. Staff were quintessentially considered to be part of a working-class culture. Officers generally held high school degrees or lower, and nurses described how they did not fit in with healthcare providers in the community. Many nurses described themselves as being both a prison officer and healthcare providers. Some staff depicted similar lived experiences to inmates, depicting overlapping social networks and comparable experiences of everyday violence. Several staff also described their prison employment as an important way out from financial difficulty or as an opportunity to access capital traditionally outside their social positions. Prison games served to create a social distinction between staff and inmates. It enabled staff to police certain morals. For example, staff sought to use prison games to generate punishment for inmates who committed certain offenses (e.g., assaulting a child or domestic violence), as well as means to uphold values such as the importance of "hard work" and contribution as American citizens.

Staff, like inmates, learned to play games through their day-to-day engagement with inmates. Their understanding and skills were different based on their level of experience; senior staff, particularly officers, were referred to as "brass", while younger staff were called "rookies". Staff shared their game playing tactics with one another orally, as well as developed a "grey code" to operate under rules not formally sanctioned by senior members of the institution. Participation in prison games was socially upheld by certain sanctions in the form of added work for those who did not play games, as well loss the of promotion opportunities and social exclusion.

Some staff, like inmates, denigrated their bodies in order to gain agency during specific situations. For example, one day I arrived at Melville reservation to set up for an exercise class in Women's Minimum. I waited in the officer breakroom for the afternoon count to clear, enabling inmates to move freely. I observed three officers as they discussed how to use prison games to secure paid time off from work. I recognised two of the officers as "bid-to-post" (those who held permanent roles in a facility and were more senior), but the third officer appeared to be visiting and was not in a uniform. One of the uniformed officers addressed the visiting officer, and said, "You lucky piece of shit, how is old Dr. Summer-off?" The man smirked and replied, "Honestly, I've had such a wonderful vacation, and my arm doesn't even hurt, you know?" The officers had discussed ways they could engineer a successful compensation claim by injuring themselves on the job. This includes instigating physical fights with inmates and intentionally slipping and falling on a wet surface. They also shared the name of a community doctor who would be sympathetic to providing them with a temporary disability status needed for validating a claim.

3.6.4 Capital

Calhoun depicts "capital" as a resource that can be immaterial, such as cultural, symbolic, and the social, as well as material or economic. It is something that ultimately yields power and agency for members in a given field (Calhoun et al., 1993, p. 69). The field of prison games and its members (inmates, officers, nurses, physicians, wardens, etc.) negotiate and compete over capital in order to maintain or improve their positions in the field (Jenkins, 2002, pp. 84–85). For inmates, capital was achieved through degrading practices, destruction and collection of material objects, and the gain or loss of freedom over time. For staff, capital was also achieved through the acts of destruction, which included inciting physical fights or destroying objects to gain control over inmates and enforce morals and ideas of the institution. Employment in prison also generated certain material and social capital indicative of a higher social status.

The next chapter, Benefits of Degradation, will explore what is at stake for inmates during prison games. It offers ethnographic detail on how inmates' destructive acts formed capital, even if only temporary, that enabled change in their social positions. First, this chapter will depict how staff and inmates view degrading behaviour differently by exploring competing notions of manipulation and agency. Next, this chapter will describe how prison games led to the procurement of certain medications in the prison setting. Attaining and destroying objects was one way inmates had control over space and time within the prison system. Finally, this chapter will introduce the concept of "intentional reimprisonment" whereby inmates return to prison, suspending certain freedoms, in order to access a site of safety and security, emotional support and hope for the future, substance detoxification, welfare and re-entry support, and paperwork for community-based benefits. Data showed that inmates who returned to prison and played prison games procured both immediate and long-term benefits within a unique marketplace predicated on violence.

References

Boston, J. (2006). *The prison litigation reform Act.* The Legal Aid Society, Prisoners' Rights Project: New York, NY. Retrieved from https://law.yale.edu/sites/default/files/documents/pdf/Boston_PLRA_Treatise.pdf.

Bourdieu, P. (1977). *Outline of a theory of practice.* Cambridge, UK: Cambridge University Press.

Bourdieu, P. (1984/2010). *Distinction: A social critique of the judgement of taste.* London: Routledge (Reprint 2010).

Bourdieu, P., & Wacquant, L. (1992). *An invitation to reflexive sociology.* Cambridge, UK: Polity Press.

Calhoun, C., LiPuma, E., & Postone, M. (1993). *Bourdieu: Critical perspectives.* Oxford, UK: Blackwell.

Christoforou, A., & Lainé, M. (2014). *Re-thinking economics: Exploring the work of Pierre Bourdieu.* New York, NY: Routledge.

Estelle v. Gamble, 429 U.S. 97, 97 426 (Supreme Court of the United States 1976).

Jenkins, R. (2002). *Pierre Bourdieu: Revised edition Richard Jenkins.* London, UK: Routledge.

Navarro, Z. (2006). Search of cultural interpretation of power: The contribution of Pierre Bourdieu. *IDS Bulletin, 37*(6), 11–22.

Thompson, J. H. (2010). Today's deliberate indifference: Providing attention without providing treatment to prisoners with serious medical needs. *Harvard Civil Rights-Civil Liberties Law Review, 45*(2), 635–654.

Wool, J. (2007). Litigating for better medical care. In R. B. Greifinger, J. A. Bick, & J. Goldenson (Eds.), *Public health behind bars: From prisons to communities.* New York: Springer.

4

Benefits of Degradation

The marketplace of prison games, a field predicated on acts of violence, was by no means free of harmful consequences for both staff and inmates, including bodily harm and death. However, one key finding from this study suggests that capital was accrued at the site of prison games. This chapter depicts how staff and inmates perceived game playing differently. It will explore agentic descriptions of degradation commonly presented by inmates. Degradation changed inmates' social positions, enabled access to resources, and engendered a perception of control over present circumstances and anticipated futures. While maintaining a focus on capital connected to inmate's health and wellbeing, this chapter will depict how certain benefits were located beyond the site of prison healthcare.

L. Kuester, *Violence in Pursuit of Health*, Palgrave Studies in Prisons and Penology, https://doi.org/10.1007/978-3-030-61350-1_4

4.1 How Do Staff and Inmates View Prison Games?

Staff and inmates viewed prison games differently, despite data suggesting that both groups deployed remarkably similar violent tactics during game playing. Staff regularly downplayed the agentic qualities of degradation, while inmates depicted this practice as imbued with capital.

4.1.1 How Staff View Prison Games

Throughout the study, staff recounted inmates' self-degradation as evidence that they were inappropriately acting entitled, manipulative, or were seeking attention. Staff depicted game playing as something that was often initiated by inmates. Typically, nurses and officers described an inmate's self-degrading behaviour as arising from boredom, frustration, resistance, or poor mental health. Nurses recounted self-degradation as a chronic nuisance, saying, "they're trying to make our job more difficult" [...] "they can't help it, they are all criminals". Collectively, staff narratives placed responsibility for prison games at the feet of inmates, and thus rendered themselves as passive victims within a game playing system. Staff also offered limited accounts in relation to structuring mechanisms of the field that might entangle themselves and inmates within the game playing practice.

The metaphor of "playing the game" was regularly used by staff. For example, Janjak, a nurse in Men's Minimum, described his day-to-day interactions with inmates by saying, "I see them, I know them, and I get ready when they come down. I love it. I love working with them, because you see them, you anticipate that they are coming to play you, and you get ready for it".

Similarly, Pep, a retired officer, illustrated how many staff saw themselves as passive "victims" during game playing, explaining:

> It is the constant games that go on. And like I said, you know, most times I can fire back and play with them. Of course, sometimes you get caught up in stuff, and it is like damn, they got me, but it is no matter how long

> you have been here, it is constant. That is why I say we are the victims, because they play this game, and they know it so well.

Linda, a nurse in Women's Maximum, also depicted a similar notion of victimisation experienced by staff during prison games, highlighting what many other nurses depicted as manipulation by offenders:

> I came here with the attitude that they were patients, and I was going to do my best to be a great nurse. I didn't realise that a lot of the time they were trying to get medications, they were trying to – a lot of the times it was lies, they were lying to me [...] I'd find out later, oh, no, I went and just re-evaluated this patient and fell for it hook, line and sinker, and I would feel stupid, really stupid.

Chapters 5 and 6 will explore prison games from the perspective of staff. The views of staff help place prison games in a shared context with inmates. Staff recounted prison games as inmate-driven behaviour intended to exploit other members of the prison, as well as take advantage of surrounding social welfare systems. Some staff described themselves as reacting to an inmate's game, depicting themselves as unwilling and passive victims. Other staff described their response to prison games as thrilling, as it enabled them to react and disrupt a sometimes monotonous day-to-day routine. Staff regularly downplayed the role of the structuring mechanisms that created and upheld a system of degradation. By shifting the responsibility of game playing to inmates, staff reinforced inmates as criminals and constructed a critical distance from their own degrading tactics when playing games.

4.1.2 How Inmates View Prison Games

Inmates accessed health and social resources through self-degradation. Game playing provided inmates with a degree of control over prison and community conditions, particularly when successfully achieving the desired outcome. Rizzo, an inmate in Women's Minimum, illustrates both common agentic qualities that arose from degradation and regular participation in prison games.

At the time of the study, Rizzo was 40 years old and had completed fifteen prison sentences for prostitution, "boosting" (theft), and possession of illicit substances. I met with Rizzo during two short sentences, as well as upon her return to the community. During the months leading up to her departure from Women's Minimum, Rizzo depicted how she went about collecting a range of benefits. At the time of her community re-entry, she described feeling optimistic because she was enrolled in specialised HIV-case management support. Case management assistance helped Rizzo apply for housing, food stamps through the Supplemental Nutrition Assistance Program (SNAP), a bus pass, and assisted with medical care provided to her through the AIDS Drug Assistance Program (ADAP). In many respects, this level of support sheltered her from participating in overt forms of degradation when playing games. However, as her story will illustrate, she was never exempt from deploying tactics of degradation, nor was she ever removed from the social field of prison games.

During one of Rizzo's HIV consultations, Dr. Goldman, an HIV specialist, referred her to the AIDS Resource Centre (ARC). This centre, developed by Drs. Goldman and McGreevy, provided HIV-positive offenders with comprehensive case management support before they departed from prison, as well as six months in the community. Rizzo reflected on this process and depicted how this support altered the field of prison games:

> A doctor is a god. They make differences in life, you know. My Doctor is my god. Their reports and their observations and their words move mountains, point-blank, point-blank.

While Rizzo was not required to engage in overt self-harming behaviour during prison games, she was nonetheless expected to demonstrate exceptional and escalating disability over time. For Rizzo, case management mitigated certain forms of self-degradation by offering an alternative pathway to capital. However, this pathway required game playing through the embodiment of a medicalised identity. According to Rizzo, this identity was nevertheless damaging, as she explained:

> They always want you on medication that says you cannot function in society without this, this, and this and this. So, therefore, the government must take care of you. Having to take meds freaks me out because, for every pill that has a side effect, there goes another pill, and before you know it, it is out of control.

I regularly observed discharge planning and case management for offenders in prison and the community. Rizzo was assigned Hillary, an ARC outreach worker, who oversaw her case. For inmates like Rizzo, access to resources was only the first step to attaining a level of capital essential to sustaining life independent from the criminal justice system. Benefits required regular returns to prison to access temporary support networks, and many inmates accepted that they would never live independently from the prison and associated benefits market.

Rizzo was well acquainted with the "re-entry industry". During one of her discharge planning meetings with Hillary, she demonstrated a comprehensive understanding of the system by generating a list of community organisation names from memory. She had memorised approximately ten charity telephone numbers, explaining:

> I have got a lot of people that I work with, even down to my probation officer. I do all the resources that are available to me. I utilise them all. I do not just know they are there, but I go in, you know, "How are you?" and "What have you got going on?".

It was exceptionally hard work for Rizzo to gain access to community benefits. I met her at the ARC shortly after her release from prison. As we moved to one of the back rooms in the centre, she pulled a ticket from a leaflet advertising free dental services, and said, "They better pay a girl if they want to pull these teeth". She went to work organising a range of potential benefits. Sitting at Hillary's desk, she phoned the Department for Children Youth and Families, inquired about free dentistry, and contacted several other organisations in order to learn about their assessment requirements. She looked up from the desk, laughed, snapped her fingers, and said, "Building networks takes a girl time you know".

Hillary identified a potential bed at a sober house, so I accompanied her and Rizzo to the initial screening appointment. Rizzo previously lived in this house and staff were familiar with her history. However, the application required candidates to retell their biographical histories upon every new application. During the screening process, Rizzo cried as the requirements of this vetting process were emotionally draining. This was by no means an easy process for Rizzo, as it involved retelling a detailed account of violent abuse, the death of her family, experience of incarceration, struggles with mental illness, substance use, and HIV-related stigma.

The housing manager ended the meeting by explaining that a bed was not currently available. Rizzo was placed on a waiting list, which required her to phone the housing manager every day at 7:00 am or she risked losing her place. She was required to undergo weekly urine and breathalyser tests, and failing to do this, or submitting a positive sample, meant that she would be disqualified from this housing. Additionally, she was required to provide evidence of continual homelessness and unemployment while waiting. Rizzo expressed her concerns about these vetting requirements:

> It is a six-month wait. What am I supposed to do for six months while you are deciding? I cannot work, because if you see that I can gather work, then I am denied automatically.

After this meeting, I drove Rizzo to a shelter on the West Side. We walked around a chain-linked fence to a low-rise cinderblock building. We stopped to share a cigarette with some residents in the parking lot before heading to the reception hall. The shelter's main room doubled as a chapel and food pantry, and the walls were covered in murals of Jesus Christ. An oversized American flag proudly hung above the registration desk. Rizzo stayed in the shelter before, and described it as unhygienic, filled with drugs, and was subject to frequent raids by police.

Obtaining benefits was hard work for persons in the criminal justice system. Rizzo explained how this process was exacerbating, and often with little reward or positive outcome, explaining, "I put in my time, I followed all the rules and went by the books. I did what they told me to do, and you think I'd get something for it, but no". Rizzo stayed homeless in order to capitalise on potential resources that never materialised.

After residing in the community for several months, she was arrested on a charge related to prostitution and returned to prison. She was disappointed, saying, "We're trying to make it the last time. Every time I go out that door, but once you go out you get slapped with reality". Rizzo depicted being caught up in a system that relied on her failure:

> You are fending for yourself; it is what it is [Melville Prison] is here to correct where I went wrong, but what are they really correcting? If they could fix everybody that comes through that door, they would not have a job. Think about the big picture. They fix one item, but there are seven more. If you fail, it keeps the prison employed.

Rizzo's quintessential journey through prison demonstrates how inmates understand prison games to be enabling of a unique claims-making process. It highlights the obstacles inmates face in procuring desired capital. Her story is representative of a group of offenders with a high-level of support, when compared to those without access to specialised HIV services. It demonstrates how prison games, and associated benefits, transcend imprisonment and into the peri-carceral space. Game playing did not always involve overt bodily destruction, but sometimes included more subtle forms of debasement, such as embodying a medicalised identity. Rizzo's account was particularly troubling, as it highlights how the benefits gained were often only temporary, of low quality, and imposed almost impossible standards for long-term support. Rizzo's story indicates how change might be momentary, or merely a feeling of hope, which ultimately ends with the return to prison and re-entry into prison games.

4.2 How Do Inmates Benefit for Prison Games?

What benefits do inmates receive from playing prison games? Game playing enabled access to a range of capital located in the prison and community. Capital enabled inmates to accrue material wealth, have more control over space and time, and shift their social positions. Access to specific treatments and therapies opened possibilities for both material goods in the prison, as well as social change upon their re-entry to the community. For example, certain medications were collected by inmates and used for trading with other inmates, often in exchange for other materials, privileges, or money. The prescription of medication also generated documentation used to support a disability claim upon their return to the community, which, in turn, opened further financial support, access to healthcare, and housing. A specific diagnosis also enabled inmates to shift their identity from that of a criminal to someone who was ill. Prison games enabled access to objects, which had capital through their destruction. Destroying objects, or one's body, was used to invoke a predictable infraction system, which enabled inmates' greater control over the amount of time would spend in prison, and where in the prison they would carry out their sentence. This chapter's proceeding sections explore different capital benefits, mapping them from prison out into the community.

4.3 Procuring Medication

Medications were widely prescribed to inmates, as this population experienced a high prevalence of communicable and non-communicable disease and mental health challenges. Certain medications, such as psychotropic drugs, functioned as trading capital among inmates because other currencies, such as money, were restricted or unavailable. Medication were delivered to inmates through *med line*, which happened twice daily at 8:00 am and 4:00 pm. Reggie, a nurse in Men's Jail, was one of the nurses who prepared medication delivery. She filled paper cups with water and arranged them on cafeteria trollies. Each housing module of inmates arrived in shifts, replenishing a long line that snaked down the hallway and up a staircase. In a small room adjoining the "chow hall" (dining facility), two nurses sat behind a chest containing pill sheets. As the nurse forced a pill from the blister, it made a distinct popping sound. Each inmate approached the delivery window, showed their I.D., and swallowed a cup of pills. Next, a duty officer would inspect each inmate's mouth to ensure they swallowed the medication.

Prison administrative documents show that during the year 2013, Melville prison spent $7.3 million on healthcare for offenders. Approximately one third, or $2.3 million, was spent on pharmaceuticals, of which $767,000 went towards the purchase of psychotropic medication. According to healthcare staff, psychotropic medications were the most common drug prescribed to inmates. It was hard to determine the exact percentage of inmates on this medication across the institution, as several facilities experienced a high turnover of residents. However, multiple nursing staff made estimates during their interviews. Nina, a nurse in Women's Maximum, claimed that "Almost all of them are on some type of psych medication". While John, a nurse in Men's Minimum, estimated that approximately 170 out of 500 inmates in the facility were on psychiatric medications. According to Reggie, a nurse in Men's Jail, approximately 350 inmates, or 35% of offenders in the facility, were on mood stabilisers at the time of the study. Dr. Cohen, a psychiatrist in Men's Jail, depicted an upward trend in the prescription of psychotropic medication, saying "When I started here, '82, years ago; right? I counted 34 inmates at first count in the total institution. Now there are about a thousand on medication".

Historically, psychotropic medication was used to control inmates. Bobby, a senior healthcare administrator, recounted how antipsychotic medication, which has a known side effect of drowsiness, was used to constrain disruptive inmates:

> I mean, it is a story I got from one of the wardens who is now retired. He told me about what he did as the lieutenant on the second shift at Maximum Security, probably during the mid-'70 s. He would get from the pharmacy a bottle of Thorazine, like a quart bottle, and every night he would pour an ounce of Thorazine in a whole bunch of glasses and fill them with orange juice. He would go down the wing and give everybody a glass, and it would stone them out for the night. That was how they kept the prison calm in those days.

At the time of the study, Bobby recognised that inmates frequently sought psychotropic medications. He described how the prescription of this medication, in part, replaced the historical practice of anaesthetising inmates, explaining:

> Somebody striking another inmate could cause a riot, which could cause serious hurt and harm to a whole bunch of people. So, I think, because medical over the years evolved into such a strong programme, we are able to treat inmates so they are quiet, because they're satisfied with the health condition of their bodies, and it works as far as keeping them calm and quiet.

Dr. Cohen, a psychiatrist in Men's Jail, depicted what medications were typically prescribed to inmates:

> The complaints go into the direction of getting the drugs they want, which is usually Klonopin. So, I give them something. And it so happens it's always a benzo. You know, lately baby coke, Seroquel. So, what they are trying to get with their complaints, you know, eventually their drug of choice.

Some inmates sought psychotropic medication to feel "numb or high" during their sentence. Patty, an inmate in Women's Maximum, described the medication side effects in this way: "When I first started coming in, I would be on medication, psych meds. Sleep, sleep, sleep. I was just numb and did nothing all day". Cam, an inmate in Men's Medium, depicted how it was not uncommon for inmates to seek medication that offered similar side effects:

> I would say 75% of the building are on psych meds. Why? Because it is a free high, or it makes you feel different. You can just go in and say "Look, I can't sleep," or "I feel like this", and it is just total bullshit.

Mental health challenges were prevalent in the prisoner population, and thus it was reasonable to expect a high proportion of inmates would require therapeutic intervention. Many inmates used their medication as it was prescribed, however, there was also substantial evidence that inmates "cheeked" desired medication, a process that involved smuggling medication through hiding it in their mouth, false teeth, the palm of their hand, etc. This was done in order to stockpile a medication so that it could be consumed in a larger quantity, thus producing an augmented therapeutic effect. Cheeking medication was the main way that it was procured for trading or sale to other inmates. Prince, an inmate in Men's Jail, described how he made a substantial profit by selling his medication in Men's Minimum:

> *Prince*: I had $100.00 worth of canteen every week. I lived like a king in here.
> *Landon*: So how do inmates pay for the medication?
> *Prince*: Well, you know, people smuggle in money. Or at Minimum you are allowed $10.00 every two weeks for the soda machines. And then work release is in the same building, and those guys get cash.

Methadone was also a highly sought-after commodity in prison. Only a handful of inmates enrolled in a research trial were given opioid replacement therapy (ORT), as the standard practice was to detox inmates upon their arrival. Warden Cook, the warden of Women's Maximum, described how inmates used sanitary pads to absorb the liquid medication and share it with other inmates. This same example was highlighted by Melville's medical director, who said:

> Lately, there has been this thing where they have been putting cotton in their mouth if they are getting liquid Methadone. They are putting the Methadone in the cotton, and then taking it out and giving it to somebody else. Which I would not have thought of [...]. There is a lot of that, it is certainly part of the problem, as it misdirects and diverts medication.

For some, their HIV-treatment altered the game playing field, as being on antiviral medication meant that would have better access to ORT, which was highly advocated by the HIV specialists. Cory, an inmate in Men's Minimum, explained:

> A lot of people are saying, "Why are you on it? And you are not in the research study" [...] It is because I am on the Atripla, which eats up the

> methadone. So, I would really-really be in severe withdrawals if I had to go up like 80 milligrams when I first started this medicine.

While cheeking medication was, in theory, often curtailed at *med line* when the duty officer inspected an inmate's mouth, it was clear that this was not always the case. Linda, a nurse in Women's Maximum, explained why cheeking medication was sometimes overlooked by staff:

> The brass [senior officers] use certain inmates for information and they get certain privileges, they are treated differently. I was told once an inmate felt she was very entitled. She had done something, like she had hoarded [stockpiled] her medication, and I was booking her, and the lieutenant told me "Don't book her". I said, "What are you talking about, don't book her?" I said "Why?" and the lieutenant said, "We use her for information". I found out at that point they get certain privileges, and they are entitled.

Medications were capital gained by inmates through prison games. The value and misdirection of certain drugs, in part, was why it was so heavily policed by staff. The medication was desired because of the psychological relief it offered inmates and the institutional order it helped to maintain. As such, medications had a value that could be traded for goods (e.g., canteen items, privileges, and sometimes cash). However, the prescription of medication also had long-term benefits outside prison. The diagnosis and treatment of specific conditions, and medical documents that accompanied a diagnosis, was used by inmates to support disability claims upon returning to the community. A disability claim, in turn, was one way that inmates could improve access to community healthcare, financial support, and housing. The long-term benefits of prescription medication will be discussed later in this chapter.

4.4 Procuring Other Objects

Everyday objects took on extraordinary meaning in prison. Prison healthcare service was one site where objects were negotiated and collected. Simple objects were often obtained through physician prescriptions and had inflated value, in part, because they were symbolic of "winning the game". Objects also served as a point of distinction for inmates. Warden Kilburn, the warden of Men's Maximum, depicted the value of everyday objects in prison:

> "You don't think I know about your [inmates] $2.00 10-year-old sunglasses, if by accident the officer drops them and steps on them, and that doesn't crush you?" I said, "Because it means nothing to me, because I can go right down the street after I leave here and buy a $2.00 pair of sunglasses and you can't. You don't think I know?"

During HIV-clinic, inmates often requested items that seemed out of place. While some requests appeared appropriate for a given course of treatment, other requests, such as extra pillows, mattresses, bunk assignments, new shoes, were collected out of a desire for distinction. Freddie, an inmate in Men's Maximum, exemplified how objects were obtained at the site of healthcare. He, like many inmates, was unsuccessful in obtaining desired objects through submitting a medical slip. However, Freddie played the system by making requests through an HIV consultant. His account represents the more subtle game playing that typically took place during clinical encounters:

> You know, I have been coming here so long that I know how to bypass the system. You will hear me say, "Don't forget my lotion" and "I want these medications changed". [...] Because you wouldn't believe what you would have to pay for lotion in the store order. Instead, I can just pay $3 for a doctor's visit and get the Lubaskin through [an HIV specialist] for free.

Nurses recognised these objects as constituting distinction in a setting where few things set them apart. John, a nurse in Men's Minimum, explained:

> It's a status symbol. If you're on a bottom bunk, you know, and usually the older guys that have been here for a while, they get bottom bunks, or some of the correctional officers' favourite inmates, "I'll put you on a bottom", you know.

Through the denial of objects, staff sought to restrict moments of power and distinction for inmates. In the case of lotion, an inmate obtaining this object was associated with pleasure, and thus, the item was restricted because it undermined the institution's punishment regime. Dotty explained, "They use the skin cream for self-pleasure [masturbation], and that's why they want the good stuff".

4.4.1 Destruction of Objects

The destruction of objects created opportunities for staff and inmates to have agency, as it enabled control over both space and time. To achieve the desired outcome, inmates would destroy a material object in place of, or in addition to, inflicting self-harm. Destruction of a material object activated a predictable infraction system, which inmates and staff played to their advantages. Warden Cook, the warden of Women's Maximum, depicted the agency that transpired through the destruction of an object, explaining, "Today's example, I find out that a female offender poured hot water and then cleanser on nesting baby birds. I am furious about that act".

Warden Cook reiterated this incident as a quintessential example of how inmates garnered agency through the use of a predictable punishment system. In Cook's example, the inmate was sent to segregation for 60 days, referred to mental health services, and received added time to her sentence. The Warden described how this inmate was unhappy about living on the wing, so segregation was one way this individual could, at least temporarily, move to a new location within the prison. Cook also described how the inmate was approaching her "good time" date, which meant she would be leaving the prison earlier than expected. Cook suspected that the inmate felt unprepared for her upcoming departure, so she might have engaged in a "bookable offense" to regain some control over the timeline of the sentence. This inmate also received a psychological evaluation, which, I suspect, generated medical documents used to support a disability claim upon her return to the community.

Staff also destroyed inmate's objects, incited fights, and sent inmates to segregation. Some staff referred to such actions as "wrecking", which was depicted by Garth, a senior health administrator:

> We go in and do cell searches. We do raids on individual cellblocks. So, you would go in there and you are searching someone's cell. Now, there's a way of doing it where you're insulting the guy, and then there's another way of doing it that you're looking for stuff, but you're not, you know, you go in and you start grabbing everything, throwing it in the air, and throwing it out the door, and ripping things, and just leaving the place a pit, and then walk out, "Nothing", and then you throw the guy back in there, he's pissed. He is really ticked off.

In this way, objects were battled over in prison. When a staff member confiscated or destroyed an object, inmates perceived this as a direct assault on their social positions. Staff's destructive actions represented a tipping point for ongoing power struggles between themselves and inmates.

During the study, several local newspapers and television programmes reported nine correctional officers and three inmates had been injured during a fight in Men's Maximum. News broadcasts showed footage of an officer being removed from the prison on a stretcher. A news presenter explained, "there are mostly bumps and bruises, although a correctional officer has a broken nose and a fractured eye-socket as a result of a clash with inmates". The Prison Director also appeared on a news programme, to explained the incident occurred when two officers approached an inmate and asked him to surrender an "unauthorised item, not a weapon, but an item he was not authorised to carry". The director explained, "the inmate refused to hand over an item, resisted handcuffing, and half a dozen inmates began to brawl".

What was this unsanctioned item, and how did it facilitate a prison brawl? The day following the event, I met with inmates Rahim and

Freddie, residents of Men's Maximum, to solicit their perspectives on what happened. Their responses illustrate how everyday objects were symbols of status and power in prison. Power relations were upheld both individually and collectively through objects. Thus, the destruction of objects by staff was understood as an extension of the destruction of self, Rahim explained:

> You know, it started with a drawing, a portrait, and the officer had grabbed the portrait and said, "You can't have it. I will hold it for you. When you are done, I'll give it to you". The officer started the situation [...]. So, the guy [inmate] said, "Yo, that's mine. You have got to give it to me. There's nothing illegal about that". Do you know what I am saying? "You've got art class in here. I had to do it for the art class, do the portrait". There has never been a problem before. [...]. And it just, an altercation started, and [the officer] was excessively forceful.

According to Rahim, the officer involved was a recent Academy graduate, a "rookie cop". He believed that the officer's actions were done to assert himself as a new "powerful player within the prison". Rahim depicted the officer as a "by the books kind of guy, an asshole, a nit-pick, someone who just wanted to pound his chest to make his dominance known".

Rahim felt that a collective response from inmates was justified in this situation. He believed it was important that officers understood "rookie cop behaviour" would not be tolerated on the wing, and inmates would act collectively to resist these kinds of actions, explaining:

> If you are going to try to degrade me for something, or try to, you know, downgrade me, do you know what I am saying? The other inmates are looking at it "Well, if the officer is going to do it to him, they're going to do it to me". You see, it is a train effect.

Freddie similarly recounted this incident and speculated on what he believes motivated the officer's destruction of an object:

> Well, it is a job. It is a job to them. The younger guys, well, the new CO's [officers] think that it's a battlefield in here [...] So the inmate said, "fuck it. Keep the fucking drawing", and the officer said, "cuff up". See

> the thing is, if you have a confrontation in here, whether that is with an officer or another inmate, these guys are bad and they come with the mace [...] it's things that are blown out of proportion [...] What the Department of Corrections fails to understand is if you treat a person with respect and dignity, you get that back. These guys [officers] are in it for the fight of their lives. Their overtime is being cut and budgets are being slashed, so you cannot blame them. Some of these guys just have got a bad-ass attitude.

Staff seizure and destruction of objects asserted their power and upheld their social position within the prison. Effectively, staff used the same infraction system to justify an inmate's movement, as well as regain control over the inmate's timeline for imprisonment. Officer White in Men's Maximum explained:

> *Officer White*: That's a tricky one, because in my opinion, if you really have enough audacity to provoke a fight with an inmate, you must have caused the initial disagreement to begin with. [...]. It is almost like you were done playing with your toy and now you just want to get rid of it.
> *Landon*: But is this something that happens a lot, or is a rare incident?
> *Officer White*: I would not say specifically it happens a lot, or that it's rare. Different situations call for different things.

Staff actions and agency will be explored further in Chapters 5 and 6. As demonstrated in the examples provided here, objects were an important agentic tool that was gained at the site of healthcare. Objects created a level of distinction for inmates, and the destruction, much like self-degradation, opened new opportunities for inmates and staff to control movement and time in prison. The structuring mechanisms of a predictable punishment system for the violation of rules turned ordinary objects into tools of agency. Agency through the destruction of objects often transcended to include benefits in the community, as object destruction compelled a psychological assessment, which, in turn, generated important medical documentation used to gain eligibility for State benefits (e.g. Social Security Disability Income; SSDI).

4.5 Returns to the Prison Marketplace

Life in the community offered criminal justice-involved persons few opportunities to live independently from the State. One interesting finding from this study was that inmates described how they frequently lowered their social standing through returns to prison over time. A temporary loss of freedom meant they could return to the prison marketplace to access certain benefits that were otherwise restricted. Patty, an inmate in women's maximum, expressed feeling overlooked in the community and depicted prison as a space she could reclaim an identity, explaining:

> In here [prison] I have a name, where on the streets people just say, 'hey you', and look right past me. I might not be always treated as a human in here, but I am definitely not respected on the streets either.

Most inmates explained how they preferred not to be incarcerated, but believed recidivism was not unexpected. Cam, a resident in men's jail, depicted how returning to the prison brought a perverse sense of stability in an otherwise unpredictable life course:

> I am pretty familiar with the system, and I know even when I get arrested, I already know what I'm kind of looking at with my record. I've been in the system like my whole life.

This sentiment was supported by his cellmate Prince, who described the prison as a disruption from the stress of everyday life, explaining:

> Out there I was working, I had to work like 50 hours a week. I'd get home, and then like I had to, you know, take a quick shower, and like rush out to an NA [Narcotics Anonymous] meeting, and then get home, and the baby don't want to go to sleep. And like by the time I get to sleep, you know, I got to be up at 5:00 in the morning. I only get five hours of sleep, and then work six days a week for one day. So, it's kind of like being in here, it's like a vacation [...].

For many, incarceration provided "time away" from community life characterised by stories of abuse, addiction, poverty, and routine encounters with the police. This was how Ricky, a man in his mid-twenties, experienced life in the community. Ricky completed five years in Men's Medium and returned to the street during the study. He was diagnosed with HIV towards the end of his sentence, and still adjusting to the health implications associated with his condition.

Ricky exited the back of a pornography shop on the West Side. I was in the area volunteering with colleagues, delivering safe injection equipment and condoms to sex workers. The shop abutted a road running parallel to an industrial estate. At night, the area was filled with young men "turning tricks". Ricky greeted me with a warm smile, grabbed my hand, and pulled me in for a hug. We walked along a chain-link fence and sat atop a barrier to talk. He was worried about his HIV and deteriorating health, explaining, "Do you see how much weight I lost? Do you remember how big I was in prison?" Ricky depicted how things fell apart after leaving prison, as he was "hit with the reality of life".

Upon leaving prison, he lived with his cousin but was soon asked to leave over a dispute about financial debt, effectively rendering him homeless. At the time of our meeting, he was facing another prison sentence connected to an outstanding warrant. In prison, Ricky was able to "lay low", but in the community, life was far more complicated. On the streets, he managed his identity differently, which was a constant source of anxiety. He kept his HIV-status and sex work secret from his girlfriend and fellow gang members. Ricky was worried that his partner would leave him, and the gang would assault him if they found out his secrets, explaining:

> I live two separate lives because, to be honest with you, you know, the other side of the streets and the other side of that bridge they know me as a gangster type; do you know what I mean?

Ricky had difficulty finding employment work because of his criminal record. He started using heroin again, saying, "it keeps me numb while

I have sex with men". A few months after this meeting, Ricky was re-incarcerated. At the intake centre within the jail, he expressed how re-incarceration meant that he could stop using drugs and get back on his antiviral medication. John, a nurse in men's minimum, suggested that Ricky's expressed relief for being re-incarcerated was not uncommon as it offered a pathway to accessing medical care:

> And we hear it all the time, "I have nobody out there". So, they go, "I need my medications. That's why I came back". "I'm homeless. I need to come back here".

4.5.1 Prison as a Place of Safety

Inmates often depicted prison as a place of security from others or oneself. Jamal, an inmate in men's maximum, explained how he viewed prison as a safe space, or at least safer than the community. He characterised his childhood by describing how his parents were incarcerated for selling crack, and he was subsequently shuffled into different foster homes. After leaving foster care, he found a sense of family with a gang. He described gang membership on one hand as constructing of a sense of belonging, but on the other hand it made it difficult for him to look after his health. Prison was a space where he could receive needed medical treatment and maintain a gang affiliation.

In addition to having HIV, Jamal required weekly furloughs to a community hospital to undergo procedures for a failing liver. While he was successful in receiving SSDI, which gave him access to medical and financial resources in the community, he still lacked the social support and safety in which to carry out treatment. Leaving prison was a source of concern for Jamal. He feared life in the community because out there he would need to perform gang duties that might put his life at risk. He felt there was no easy way to detach himself from the gang. He explained how to leave the gang he would need to endure a "beat-out" that would involve a physical assault from other gang members. Jamal described what prison meant for him:

> I can more or less get my head clear in here, because the people out there is like when I don't want them around, they come around, and it's kind of hard to get away from them. [...] When I get out, I'm going to gang-bang even harder, and probably that's going to lead to be getting hurt really bad, or, do you know what I'm saying? - like just dying.

Martin, an inmate in men's medium, similarly depicted prison as a site for security and access to care. He described a psychiatric hospital as the only other place where he felt safe and could plan for his future and work on his mental health issues. Since he couldn't afford long-term hospital treatment, he explained how he would return to prison when things got too difficult. He depicted how the therapy groups, staff in the hospital made him feel like he was somebody and had hope for a better future, explaining:

> [Family member] actually caught me with a gun in my mouth, then I had one to my head [...]. So, I end up going into [psychiatric hospital]. I tried hanging myself. I overdose on my pills a lot, I will do that a lot. [...]. And then once I started using the drugs, I wanted to stop so bad, but it was like I couldn't find a way to stop [...] The only time I actually felt comfortable, when I felt like shit could change, was when I was put in [psychiatric hospital].

Both prison and the psychiatric hospital had the same effect of removing Martin from a violent life in the community, while simultaneously providing him with greater opportunities to collect resources and experience care. He explained how, shortly after release from the hospital, he committed a crime to re-enter the correctional setting in order to continue to have some level of support.

4.5.2 Emotional Support and Hope for the Future

Incarceration provided a routinised way of living with reduced responsibility, which enabled time to devote to oneself. Prison also offered relief from the stress of HIV-related stigma, which was most pronounced when pursuing relationships in the community.

For Patty, prison became a space for her to work on her emotional wellbeing. Now in her thirties, she has completed over a dozen prison sentences. During our discussion she unfolded a biographical history, which included being raped as a young teen and becoming pregnant. Patty started using crack in her twenties, and shortly after started engaging in sex work to support her drug habit. She described how she viewed regular visits to prison like a "saviour" not only from physical health risks associated with illicit substance misuse and precarious nights on the street, but for the space it provided for her to hope and plan. She described how this hopeful outlook was only something she experienced when incarcerated. She articulated that it was "time" that allowed her to imagine a new future:

> You think like what else can happen to me, other than die? When you're so enmeshed in that lifestyle, sometimes I would rather something happen to me than keep doing what I was doing, but it was all I knew how to do. The worst would never happen, so I was just scathing it. But to come to prison or to get arrested, sometimes it was like a saviour. Sometimes it was like thank God, like, I got arrested. [...]
>
> Here you know what's next. Out there, when you don't have nowhere to go, you don't have family, you don't have the support, you don't know what's next. You have to make next [...] So you have to be responsible for yourself. Not that you don't have to be responsible for yourself here, just here you're guided.

Patty mostly resided on parole in the community for the duration of the study. With assistance from her case manager, money from a minimum wage job and welfare benefits, she secured housing, opened a bank account, and filled her refrigerator with food. Like many other inmates living with HIV, she described how life was difficult because it was her first time having romantic relationships and being HIV-positive, and as a result she felt increasingly isolated. After several months of living in the community, Patty surrendered herself to a parole officer and returned to prison. She knowingly violated her parole conditions by having a few alcoholic drinks, and said it was because she felt lonely, overworked, and was burnt out.

Prison was a place where inmates avoided complicated relationships and stigma. This was also the case for Johnny, an inmate in Men's Jail, who spent most of his adult life in prison. Jonny used drugs to cope with the emotional pain he experienced in the community, explaining:

> I fell in love, after having courted her for some time. She began to speak of marriage, children, and a future together. Tears poured down my face. I stopped to pick up some dope and a set of works to ease my pain. Hitting myself in the darkness, a single question would pop into my head; what have you got to lose anyway? […] It is how I dealt with this kind of pain and loss.

Prison offered Johnny a choice. He could either live on the street where reality was messy, erratic, and dangerous, or return to prison so that he would not "lose it all and die". He depicted his mental state leading up to his imprisonment:

> I had lost my will to live. My life no longer had meaning nor purpose. What was the point of going on? No kids, no wife. I did not really care if someone put an end to it all for me, as I no longer wanted to go on living in pain and misery. I spent years medicating myself. Drugs served a real purpose. My fears, my pain, my guilt would all vanish by simply escaping reality.

Prison presented a different kind of escape, one where Jonny could receive medication for depression, stop using drugs, and avoid stressful relationships. In many respects, Jonny was institutionalised, reliant on the support that prison offered, and felt unable to navigate the stress of everyday life in the community:

> Nobody prepared me for these types of issues outside prison. Protective measures where are all I was taught […]. If I did not get arrested that day, I am afraid I would have taken an overdose of heroin and died.

4.5.3 A Place to Detox

Inmates and ex-inmates who struggled with drug dependence often viewed incarceration as a positive biographical disruption from addiction. Rob, an inmate in men's jail, described prison as a space that saves lives by removing people from certain conditions and risk behaviour associated with substance misuse in the community:

> Being incarcerated again […] forced me to stay clean; do you know what I mean? I can't take that from the system at all. […] Sometimes I feel like, you know, this place saves people's lives.

Junior, the son of an inmate in men's medium, further described how he accessed drug detoxification and treatment through entering the prison system. He explained that from age twelve he sold heroin with his father to make a living. He grew up in a context where dealing and using drugs was considered normal. He explained that prison provided him with regular opportunities to detox, and to receive referrals to community-based drug treatment programmes upon release. However, his access to community treatment was only temporary and required regular returns to prison to maintain his programme enrolment at reasonable cost. Junior expressed his desire to break this cycle of drug use and regular returns to prison, but could not identify a suitable alternative:

> My father just said to me earlier today -- "we will never be okay out here because out here you know you can get it" -- when my girl leaves me in the morning and I've tried to hide from her. I cry and think 'if I get too deep this time, I'm going to lose everything. I have got to get myself a little bit of time to sober up. I've got to get another voucher. How do I get a voucher without going to prison?'

4.5.4 Welfare and Re-Entry

Re-entry programmes support inmates in securing housing, medical care, substance addiction support, and other benefits. Some inmates expressed a desire to return to prison to access re-entry programmes. Freddie, an inmate in Men's Maximum, when discussing his experience with ARC, depicted a need for intensive case management support to remain in society. He described how when time sensitive support was about to end, he would return to prison to become eligible for continued case management:

> I go to places like [ARC] because they are there. You know, this is a good programme, I was one of the first people to be a part of it, and they aren't getting rid of me (laughing) -- and then I come to jail -- but here's the thing, it is supposed to be a 6 month programme and every time I got near the 6 months I'd come back to jail. I'd come back to jail just so I could get back into the programme.

For many inmates, the re-entry journey was marked by little or no support, but for others the process extends for years after release through lengthy parole conditions. Inmates consistently described needing better re-entry support, and explained that existing programmes often had poor oversight, were too short, and inconsistent due to funding variations. Nevertheless, inmates interviewed during the study, exemplified by Freddie and Junior, presented a growing narrative expressing how they might intentionally return to prison to gain access to re-entry resources.

Hillary, a caseworker with ARC, described how accessing appropriate community welfare took years, and was impossible for inmates to obtain given their often-complex financial and social situations. She depicted how it was not uncommon for an ex-inmate's assistance to terminate prior to obtaining long-term support, explaining:

> There is a big myth about how easy it is to get SSI [Social Security Income]. But SSI is extremely hard to get, it's like winning the jackpot. It takes about two years. You get rejected twice, and only on the third application, you go in front of a judge with hired legal counsel and make a case for why you should receive support. Many of our clients become re-incarcerated during this process, which causes further delays. The pathetic part of it all is, that you only get $714.92 per month. This is not enough to support you on the street. I could not do it […] they have restitution to pay, child support, health costs, housing and, often a drug addiction […]

4.5.5 Building Medical Records

Receiving a diagnosis in prison and being prescribed medication was critical for inmates to have a chance at obtaining community benefits. This medical intervention shifted their identity from criminal too ill. A range of prison members explained the role of medical documentation in their disability diagnosis, a key component of the eligibility criteria for SSI and SSDI.

This was the focus of my discussion with an ex-inmate, Casper, who I met in his small, white 1920s Roebuck style home on the outskirts of Melville. Casper, who had completed a six-month ARC programme many years ago. He had been in and out of prison since the late 1970s, adding up to about twenty-five years inside prison. Casper's SSI welfare was terminated when he was incarcerated. He elucidated how having access to healthcare in prison provided him with an opportunity to create a medical record for completing a successful SSI application. He expressed how obtaining SSI was a lengthy process that commenced in prison and continued with community-based organisations after release. He also described how both his HIV-positive status and mental health diagnosis were important medical conditions for making a strong case for receiving welfare, explaining:

> Yeah, you share that [share information with other inmates], you know, like saying, "Well, you know, you got to go see the psych doctor, you know, and tell him that, you know, like you're depressed, or you know, you're suicidal", and all of that stuff. So, each time you're saying all this stuff, they're writing things down; And certain things, they give you medicine for it; do you know what I mean? Now you got a paper trail. […]

Prison nurses described Casper's pursuit as a common pathway to welfare support, and along with administrators highlighted different features of this practice. Allen, a nurse in men's minimum explained how it was not uncommon for sick inmates to "play up" their medical symptoms to become eligible for a disability diagnosis, he explained:

> It's kind of hard, because a lot of people -- I mean, we have a lot of sick people, really sick, but then we have a lot of people that they do fake the sickness, because a lot of people are there, and they want to be out in society. When they get out of prison, they like to collect cheques. Their goal is like "Well, if I'm in prison on any medication, then I have support to say, well, I'm bipolar". They want to be diagnosed with anything that will qualify them to get a cheque every month.

Another nurse in men's jail explained how inmates might continue to pursue a disability diagnosis after prison, however, suspected many of them never took prescription medications in the community. Bobby, a senior healthcare administrator, explained how an inmate's HIV diagnosis was no longer sufficient for SSI and SSDI eligibility. He identified how the introduction of antiviral medication led to a higher rejection rate of claims in recent years. This meant that inmates living with HIV would need further documentation, something that could be achieved through degradation in prison, to receive a diagnosis that might meet the standards of a disability (Appendix D: Welfare & Medical Benefits). Donnie, an inmate in Men's Minimum, explained how resources for people living with HIV have dissipated:

> A lot of things have changed. Like in the beginning, I see a lot of things happening. I would say like '97, '98, '99, I seen a lot of people getting in housing, you know, getting a lot of help just because of the [HIV] funds. And a lot of funds have ran out, and they are not getting funded no more. I mean we don't get nothing now.

This chapter has depicted several benefits inmates can gain through re-entering imprisonment and playing prison games. It highlights the benefits that were produced through the structuring mechanisms of imprisonment and social welfare systems, which favours the reproduction of degradation during prison games. The next chapter will consider prison games from the experience of staff, including perspectives from nurses, officers, wardens, healthcare practitioners and other employees of the prison. Staff understand and manage prison games in relation to their own social worlds, morals, and values. Staff members attempt to present themselves as socially distinct from inmates, despite having similar biographical experiences in the community and prison. This leads some staff to actively degrade inmates to police social boundaries between themselves and inmates within a shared environment, determining who was deserving of care.

5

The Staff Who Play Prison Games

At the time of this study, Melville prison employed over 1,400 people. Divisions of labour included a director's office and administration, correctional industries, institutional operations, media and community relations, probation and parole services, rehabilitation services, and victims' services.

Prison administration comprised 90 employees and an assistant director that worked "behind the scenes". This division retained staff in a diversity of roles, including finance, human resources, information management, planning and research, policy, and officer training. Staff services included payroll, recruitment, labour relations, and processing of injury claims. Services for inmates included management of financial accounts, commissary, mail and courier services, and management of offender data. There was in-house IT support. Planning and research worked on both short-and-long-term programme development, while policy staff ensured that department-level protocols were in line with applicable rules, regulations, statutes, and national standards. An officer training academy ran a nine-week prison officer accreditation course and provided in-service training to all staff.

L. Kuester, *Violence in Pursuit of Health*, Palgrave Studies in Prisons and Penology, https://doi.org/10.1007/978-3-030-61350-1_5

Correctional industries relied on inmate labour to produce "prisoner-made goods" sold to state agencies and non-profit organizations. Industries employed shop and contract supervisors, as well as civilian administrative staff that reported to an associate director. From 2011–2013, correctional industries had an average revenue of $2,175,331. Workstreams included the production of clothing, furniture, manufacturing of licence plates, and printing, as well as services that included cleaning, landscaping, removals, and painting. Offenders were compensated $0.50 to $3.00 per day for work.

Institutional operations comprised a workforce of approximately 933 correctional officers in charge of custody, control, and the movement of inmates. There were emergency response and crisis intervention teams. Operations also employed staff to oversee building maintenance, food services, and a team overseeing the investigation of all alleged inmate misconduct.

Rehabilitation staff offered healthcare services, transitional and discharge programming for offenders leaving prison, and delivered some aspects of community corrections. Staff delivered educations services, vocational training, library services, and chaplaincy. Rehabilitative staff were also responsible for offender classification. Inmate healthcare was overseen by a medical director, healthcare administrator, and director of nursing. Healthcare services were supported by administrators and record keeping. Medical services were delivered by behavioural and mental health professionals, dentists, general practitioners, HIV consultants, 43 licenced nurses, physician assistant, and a public health specialist nurse.

Probation and parole services were responsible for offenders and community-based correctional supervision. There was a parole board, 79 probation and parole Officers, 9 supervisors, a deputy administrator, and 24 support staff. Probation and Parole was managed by an administrator and an assistant administrator reporting to an associate director.

Prison officers and nurses were considered frontline staff. Nursing staff held dual titles of correctional officer and nurse. Security staff followed a militarised ranking system which, in ascending order, included the ranks of Warden, Deputy Warden, Captain, Lieutenant, and Correctional Officer. Informally, new officers were referred to as "rookie cops", while senior officers were designated as "bid to post", which meant they had the right to select their positions within a prison facility. Ranking senior officers were referred to as "Brass".

This chapter will explore prison games from the standpoint of staff, focusing on employees who worked on the frontline. The staff provided similar biographical narratives to inmates, and both groups "did time" together in the same prison environment. Despite having uniforms and the ability to come and go from the correctional setting, staff played games to their benefit, policed moral boundaries, and created a distinction between themselves and inmates.

The prison work culture was conducive to staff playing prison games. Officers described immature and childish behaviour, younger staff felt unprepared to police inmates, and "hard work" was understood through contact with inmates and playing games. Staff, in part, degraded inmates to distance themselves from offending behavior, while at the same time reinforcing inmates' social positions as "less deserving" when compared to themselves and other law-abiding citizens. Thus, staff co-produced a marketplace of violence with inmates.

5.1 Inmates and Staff Are Alike

5.1.1 Staff Experience in the Community

Staff depicted similar biographical experiences to inmates. Staff accounts distinguished their personal and professional lives as being somewhat different from members of the public. When describing challenges in their personal and professional lives, they depicted how other members of society "just didn't get it", while at the same time acknowledging that their experiences brought them closer to inmates. Staff and inmates came from the same neighbourhoods, and both groups ended up in prison, albeit in different roles.

Gina, a nurse in Men's Jail, recounted growing up in the same community as many inmates:

> I grew up in [South Melville]. I grew up right off [street name], and I used to hang off [street name]. You know, I have been beaten up by black

> guys. I thought they were going to rape me. They fucked me up good. Dragged me around the corner. Oh, yes, I thought I was dead. They must have been getting high or something. And I was like "Oh, my God" [...] so, growing up like that helps me relate to them [inmates].

Gina's experience of violence and insecurity was relived through her memories, which, in turn, informed her understanding of the offender population. However, her personal engagement with this violence and the offending community was not just located in the past. Gina, like other members of staff, depicted a common challenge of delivering services to friends or family who were incarcerated:

> Now, the guy that raped my cousin's daughters, he was married to my cousin, comes into sick call while I'm at Medium, and he rolls up his sleeve, and on his arm, it says "[cousin's name]". That is my cousin, that is the one he married. And I am looking at this guy and like I want to like pop him [...]. I look at him, and I try not to think about it. But if I were to sit there and think about it, I would stick my high heel in his eyeball, you know.

This intersecting social network was also depicted by senior staff. Warden Kilburn, the warden of Men's Maximum, explained that an overlapping social network between inmates and staff was the unique result of a prison system that served a local community, explaining:

> I walk the blocks; I walk the tiers. I will go to the dining room. They can write to me. Their family members -- you see, [Melville] is unique. It is not unusual for somebody like me to go into the cell block and see somebody I went to school with, see a neighbour, see a relative, see the son of an inmate that I had before, or a grandson. And it is not unusual for a phone call from a concerned mother about her son, that recognises my name and asks me where my family came from, and they went to school with my mother or my father.

While staff commonly depicted difficulties that resulted from having personal connections to the prisoner population, others described how their shared biography made them more empathetic towards the many challenges inmates typically faced in their lives. For example, Officer White, an officer in Men's Maximum, described how personal struggles with addiction enabled her to be more compassionate to inmates in a similar position, explaining:

> My difference is that I take into consideration that they are people and not caged animals, and that is the difference. And a lot of people, a lot of officers do not get trained to do that. It is the difference between, you know, clinical and substance abuse counsellors and an officer. We get trained to be hard-core, take anything.

Officer Lazzeri, an officer in Women's Maximum, also depicted a similar experience to Officer White when describing her empathy for inmates going through substance detox:

> I have got a brother that is going through some hard times right now. I totally understand the addict. I have got it in my family. I think officers are in a false sense. I think they put themselves up whether they have the problem or not. They already feel one up, so they have already separated themselves from them, where for me I know that it is just a hairline away from my own experience.

Officer Lazzeri's narrative is telling for what it reveals about staff who actively degrade inmates. The staff did not want to recognise themselves as being the same as inmates. Doing so eroded a critical distance between themselves and the offending population. Acknowledging empathy meant staff would have to come to terms with their role in perpetuating violence within a group of people like themselves, a practice that would be easier to do if they were understood inmates as being other, or "criminal".

Warden Cook, the warden of Women's Maximum, explained why staff adopted a "tough guy" demeanour, particularly when interacting with inmates. She described how dozens of officers secretly sought her support for "depression, suicidal thoughts, and alcoholism". Cook said that "the stress of the job really takes a toll, and people just struggle to cope". She believed many staff members suffered in silence out of fear that they would be seen as weak or unfit for duty. Cook also articulated what I observed during ethnographic observations: staff who appeared to suffer mentally, and those who had closely shared biographies with inmates, were most likely to actively degrade inmates. Samantha, the deputy director of Rehabilitation Services, provided an example of a staff member who struggled with depression and was known to engage in actively degrading behaviour:

> Well, I had a correctional officer when I was the warden over there. She was just my nemesis. I would hear stories from the inmates, "You don't know what she did. Last night she made me clean the floor with a toothbrush". She [officer] ended up killing herself, committing suicide.

5.1.2 Doing Time Together

Staff depicted how they were "doing time" with inmates. It was not uncommon for staff to describe working overtime shifts on top of lengthy schedules, leading one nurse to explain, "I'm here so much, I feel like I just go home on work release. We're doing time on an installment plan". Historically, there was no limit to staff overtime, as Mark, a nurse in Men's Medium, recounted:

> Well, the record is a full week. One person stayed here for seven straight days. It used to be years ago they did not allow nursing pools in here. So, any given time it is like "Hey, Mark, guess what? You are working 3:00 to 11:00 tonight. And then after you finish the 3:00 to 11:00 shift, guess what? 11:00 to 7:00. And then guess what? 7:00 to 3:00". It was my longest, eight shifts.

Mark described the potential health consequences of working consecutive shifts. He, like other staff, worried about losing their job if they refused to carry on working:

> If you didn't want to work, you'd lose your job. Or get suspended, or something like that. But, you know, it is at any given time. At the end of the eight shifts I told them [Nursing Director], I said "Listen, I can't

> see straight. I mean, I am not safe, you know, you have got to let me go. I've got to get some sleep".

An inmate's self-degradation during prison games generated more work for staff, as it required their attention and completion of incident reports. An inmate's self-degradation meant staff would have less "dead time" to cope with the exhaustion of working long shifts. It also meant that staff were often delayed in leaving the prison. Linda, a nurse in Women's Maximum, explained:

> By the time I finished giving a report, so many people are, you know, under duress, and are in segregation, and they all want to hurt themselves. And count all the sharps and all the medications, narcotics. And then by the time you get home, you have got four hours to sleep, and then you are back up. It feels like you never left.

This scenario led staff to resent inmates who self-degraded, which sometimes provoked them to respond by actively degrading inmates or withholding medical care. Reggie, a nurse in Men's Jail, described how this situation generated frustration towards inmates:

> You can see people who do a lot of overtime, you can see it in their faces. You know, you see them age. You have no patience for the inmates. You do not want to see another inmate. You do not want to hear, you do not care, and that is not healthy.

Staff who spent extended periods in prison developed inappropriate personal relationships with inmates. Officer White, an officer in Men's Maximum, depicted how staff gained intimate knowledge of inmates lives over time:

> It becomes like you live with these people. I could tell you right now what religion they are, how many kids they have, boy or girl, if they are married, how many baby mommas they have. I can tell you what their annual income is, I can tell you how many cars they drove or have, what their trade outdoors is, what their schedules are. I can tell you who is going to go on a visit, what day, who is not. And that is just from being

> in the same block for one year. That is one year. Imagine the officers who have been in the same building or in the same block for a long time.

Officer White, along with several wardens, depicted how close relationships between staff and inmates often crossed legal and social boundaries. They provided several accounts where staff and inmates had sexual relationships. This finding was particularly worrying because of the power differentials under conditions of imprisonment. However, such accounts further elucidated the fragile social boundaries between inmates and staff, as well as explain why staff might degrade inmates to construct a critical distance.

Inmates depicted sexual relationships with staff as another site of prison games. Damian, an inmate in Men's Minimum, described a sexual encounter with a staff member in medical records, which took place in the past. He viewed his sexual relationship with a member of staff as an opportunity to improve his social position upon leaving the prison:

> It is funny because she worked in [medical records]. So, she already knew about my HIV status. I did corner her down there one day, you know, and snuck a kiss, and you know. One thing led to another, and when I got out, and she offered, you know, to move me into her home. She had that job, she had her own apartment, and she just got a new car. So, honestly, it was very accommodating. I am not going to lie. I was in jail nine years. I mean shave a dog down, I would have probably, do you know what I am saying? A year later we got married.

Staff depicted burnout that resulted from their professional work, which had detrimental consequences on their personal lives. Garth, a healthcare administrator, identified how stressful working conditions led to a high number of relationship breakdowns for himself and his colleagues:

> I'm trying to think of who's married and who's not. I mean, a lot of us have been divorced at least once, almost all of us. Most of us are single. We are a product of our environment, and by working with these inmates you become argumentative; we are like professional arguers. You argue with every guy in *Med line*. Every guy that comes up.

5.1.3 A Sheared Dependency on Imprisonment

Staff, like inmates, recognised prison as a site for gaining capital that was typically outside their social position. Prison officers were required to have a high school diploma or general education diploma (GED) and complete a nine-week training course. Nurses were required to have a high school diploma or GED and complete nursing education training, which was generally achieved through earning a certificate or diploma from an approved nursing programme.

In 2013, the average salary for an equivalent education was $30,000 (National Center for Educational Statistics, 2014). However, prison staff exceeded the national average through accruing overtime pay. Overtime compensation, negotiated through a strong employment union, enabled staff to accrue substantial wealth. Public records showed that during 2013, prison and nursing staff earned up to $200,000 per year.

For example, Gina, a nurse in Men's Jail, earned over $124,000 in the fiscal year 2013, far exceeding the $40,000 to $46,000 she would expect to earn in a community healthcare setting. Gina, like other staff, depicted how her employment in prison meant that she could pay off debts as well as purchase property. However, she also described a common sentiment of feeling financially dependent on the prison as a way out from debt, explaining:

> I feel like I hit the lottery when I finally got the job. I was like "Way cool", you know. But I do not give a rat's ass. The building could burn around me. I am making my money and I am leaving it all behind.

Mark, a nurse in Men's Medium, and Officer White, an officer in Men's Maximum, depicted financial decisions that underpinned common decisions to work overtime:

> *Mark*: For me it is the money, bottom line. I mean, we all have reasons. I have got another college education to pay for, so that is why I work. I do not want my kids to have a million loans.
>
> *Officer White*: You have guys that work quads all the time, "Oh, I've got to buy a new truck, I've got to buy a new car". They are not coming into do their job, they are coming into make some money.

Working for the prison was a State job, which also meant employees were also eligible for retirement packages upon completing service. Many staff expressed how this financial incentive motivated them to seek employment from the prison and stay in their jobs for extended periods. Pep, a retired prison officer, and Dotty, a nurse in Men's Jail, exemplified this common incentive:

Pep: Like most people, what attracted me to it was a pension. Like wow, that sounds pretty good. At the time I had started, free healthcare, you know. […]. And then it was like do you know what? You can make a pretty good living here, too. If you don't mind working some overtime.

Dotty: Well, what keeps me here is simply the time in service. I am right now 28 years into a pension.

Staff often described inmates as the raw human capital keeping prisons in operation, and thus keeping them employed. Warden Cook, the warden of Women's Maximum, and Dr. Cohen, a psychiatrist in Men's Jail, explained:

Warden Cook: So, what happens is, you know when something happens. I mean, some horrific crime gets committed, I can go "Oh, job security". And even though I find it appalling, I cannot dwell on it, because the people I work with have all, many have committed that, or a similar crime.

Dr. Cohen: The officers are very conscious of that. You know, when I come in the morning and I look at the board and say, "That's quite a board, 12 people on suicide watch", the officer says, "Job security". You know, so they are very much aware of the fact that the prisoners keep them employed.

Inmates were also aware of their role in the prison economy and often described how the correctional staff "worked for them", as Marco, an inmate in Men's Medium, and Freddie, an inmate in Men's Maximum described:

Marco: Anybody that commits a crime, they think they should be here. It is job security. I mean, they want their job security, because they want to make their exorbitant salaries and get paid.

Freddie: This here is [prison] business, and it is sad to say. It is all about job security for these guys. Prison has an obligation to society. If you send a man out with no hope, he is bound to come back. Here it is, when you leave [prison], you go in front of a judge [referring to parole] and say "your honour, I can't find a job" and he says "well, let's put you back in jail for a month and we'll bring you back on such and such a date" [...] The fact is people need to survive and you have to provide a way for people to survive.

5.1.4 The Staff Who Self-degrade

Chapter 3 of this book mentions that staff, like inmates, engaged in self-degradation in order to gain access to certain rights and resources. This was a particularly interesting research finding, as it highlighted the structuring mechanisms of the prison, which left no one untouched when it came to the playing of prison games. This finding also helps to explain why staff often refused to recognise the agentic qualities underpinning self-degradation for inmates, as doing so would be an admission of the fragile separation between themselves and offenders. It acknowledges that inmates held little reasonable choice but to engage in violence when pursuing rights and resources.

Structural degradation, imposed through prison rules and regulations, often left staff with few options to control aspects of their livelihood, safety, and well-being. This meant that staff entered a marketplace of violence in order to protect their positions and capital. For example, pregnant officers were not entitled to maternity leave, and thus they engaged in self-degradation to remove themselves from risky situations. While staff recognised that it was unsafe for pregnant women to be working on the frontline, they also referred to institutional policy that restricted pregnancy from warranting compensated leave or transfer to "light duty". Dean, a prison training officer, explained:

> We have been wrestling with that issue [pregnancy] up here. It may sound chauvinist, whatever, but as a female officer here you might want to make sure you have outside insurance, because pregnancy does not get you light duty and it isn't counting as a disability.

Officer White, an officer in Men's Maximum, was pregnant at the time of the research. She described participating in self-degrading behaviour in order to receive light duty during a high-risk pregnancy. She had a fellow officer drop a stack of metal trays on her head from a second-tier landing in Men's Maximum. White believed that an injury to the head would be far enough away from her pregnant belly. By inflicting this injury, she explained that she was able to make a claim for a work-related disability:

> We do it no matter what. If life has come up with a brick wall, what do you do? You have got to figure out a way around it. If there is something important that needs to go on in your life, what do you do? Do you lose your job, do you take a risk, or do you just slip and fall; do you know what I mean?

There was also some evidence that staff also shared different strategies for self-degrading tactics, which they used to play against the system. There were reports of a well-established "code" developed by staff, as Officer Rodgers, an officer in Women's Maximum, described:

> A grey code. Oh yeah, they have like signs for like the lieutenant, for the captain and they do sniper calls and they call each other down the block. You know, because in most of the buildings they must go from one area of the building to the next. So, they will call and say, "so and so just left". There is nowhere to hide in here, there are just cameras everywhere. Even the voice, once you push the button it activates it in the control centre so that they can hear everything you are saying.

5.2 How Does the Prison Structure Affect Staff?

Institutional rules and procedures shape the field of prison games for everyone under its remit. However, the "work culture" of imprisonment impacted staff differently. Staff described an immature prison workforce, "bid to post" policy that determined who was exposed to inmates, and lacking oversight and supervision from Brass. These factors were just some of the conditions that enabled a culture of violence where prison games became "hard work" for staff.

5.2.1 A "High School" Work Culture

Warden Cook, the warden of Women's Maximum, depicted how staff used immature and crude language when speaking with one another:

> It's the only business in the world where you can walk into the staff break room before roll call starts, and somebody looks up at you, and you can say, "What the fuck do you want?", and they say, "What the fuck do you care?"

Cook explained that the use of vulgar language was the equivalent of putting "little shock bombs" in everyday conversation. Staff used profanity to signal their "aggression", or as Cook elaborated, "I'm saying fuck you in a nice way, but I can lay down if I've got to, you know". The language that the staff used is telling for what it reveals about their aversion to showing softness and compassion towards others. It was important for staff to be seen as "hard", so thus the use of profanity was one way to gain this credibility and establish a sense of camaraderie among their fellow officers.

Multiple staff depicted a professional culture equivalent to "high school". Staff described long stretches of boredom, particularly on night shifts, punctuated by unpredictable moments of total chaos. Warden Cook, the warden of Women's Maximum, and Officer White, an officer in Women's Maximum, represented the professional milieu as being immature:

> *Warden Cook*: It is junior high school. I had a situation wherein one of the buildings I worked in, we were shipping almost half of our population to another building so we could complete renovations. So, we just kind of doubled up. The six months the officers were doubled up and tripled up on their post, my sexual harassment and discrimination cases quadrupled, because they were bored, they had nothing to do, so they picked on each other.

Officer White: In high school, you spend eight hours a day together. You know people. We sit at night for eight hours, we watch movies together, and we talk about stuff together, or we play games together. [...] And for eight hours of the day, they're [officer] my husband, they're pretty much, because they're looking out for me, you know, they're feeding me, they're taking care of my well-being, you know. It becomes like—you know, and then you must draw boundaries, because then it gets too much, it gets too much.

Officer White also illustrated a common challenge that female officers faced in a male-dominated profession, explaining that she and her fellow female officers were often pressured to have sex with male officers and Brass:

They [officers] meet in the gas station at night, overnight, and use their hour for whatever they are going to do. [...] It stems from the fact that they have created relationships beyond officer-to-officer, and now they are sleeping together [...] Brass are included. There have been some people who told me, you know, women get positions because of stuff that they do, wardens and brass and stuff. I mean, it gets fishy.

The staff social culture was framed by profanity, childish behaviour, sexual harassment, and sexual misconduct. The notion of the prison workplace as "high school" illustrates how staff often acted like immature youth, pushed the boundaries of socially acceptable behaviour, and tested if alternative rules and allowances would be tolerated in the prison environment.

5.2.2 Prison Games Are Hard Work

For staff, prison work was defined by routine daily tasks. Nurses reviewed medical slips, delivered medication to inmates, carried out diabetic tests, consulted inmates and physicians, performed ex-rays, counted sharps, stocked medications, called the pharmacy, and filled out paperwork. Officers conducted count, maintained order, walked the perimeter, operated security doors, oversaw visitation, escorted inmates within the facility and to outside appointments, and also filled out paperwork. These work tasks structured their workday, however, "hard work" in prison happened when staff encountered unforeseen challenges, chaos erupted, or they played prison games with inmates.

Staff sought to distance themselves from prison games by "bidding-to-post", which meant they would select a facility, role, and work shift that minimised daily contact with inmates. "Bidding" was a process afforded to senior staff through negotiations with the prison union, which offered staff considerable autonomy over their day-to-day work. High-security facilities had limited movement and reduced contact with inmates, while Jail's and low-security facilities had more turnover and required more contact with offenders. Nina, a nurse in Women's Maximum, which also functioned as a Jail, and Ritchie, a nurse in Men's Supermax, portrayed the contrasting prison environments:

> *Nina*: I work days in [Women's Maximum]. It's a huge turnover. That is the complicated part of this building. You have people that come in over the weekend, and without their medications, mostly have got in a scuffle, or stab their boyfriend, or missed a court date. You check on their medications; you work with the psychiatrist; you work with the medical doctors. You deal with trauma, you deal with infection, you deal with pregnancy, you deal with all these people […] I feel like I work in an emergency room.
>
> *Ritchie*: I work days in [Men's Supermax]. So, for me this is perfect at this point in my career. I will not be running around like at [Men's Jail], where there were—we have them here, too, but it is lower-key […].

Staff understood "hard work" as something that was determined through contact with inmates and the playing of prison games. Reggie, a nurse in Men's Jail, drew this distinction by explaining, "It is just too much here [Men's Jail]. They are always trying to get something off you. You are always getting played. And you are busy".

Earlier in this Chapter, Officer White, an officer in Men's Maximum, described how a typical nightshift involved safety checks, movies, talking, and playing games. Nights were a time when close relationships with colleagues were established, and there was less interaction with inmates. However, the trade-off for working evenings meant that staff spent less time with family and friends during social hours. Allen, a nurse in Men's

Minimum, depicted how slow-paced evening shifts would come to life in the morning:

> You deal with the doctors in the morning, they are busy. At [Men's Jail] we get commitments every single day. We get commitments all day long. So, by the time you come in in the morning, there are a lot of people that need to be taken care of. It is much busier.

Staff on different shifts were often at odds with one another. Gina, a nurse in Men's Jail, described how staff would "pass off work" in order to limit their contact time with inmates, she explained:

> That is the complacency that I was telling you about that I see frequently. And a lot of times I come in and I go "Whoa, like we have a task nurse. What do you mean I have to do this?" If you have a nurse that does the tasks or treatments, you have a treatment nurse on 7:00 to 3:00, why are those treatments being passed on to 3:00 to 11:00.

Passing off work resulted in the active degradation of inmates and had harmful health consequences. It meant that treatment would be delayed, as John, a nurse in Men's Minimum, explained:

> I am off Friday and Saturday. I had an inmate come to a nurse on Thursday night saying, "I can't see out of my right eye"; "Go see John on Sunday". The guy lost his vision. They said, "If he was brought to us within 24 hours, we would have saved his vision".

Passing off tasks meant that some staff would be more exposed to prison games, and thus they would need to work harder at their jobs. Inmates also knew which staff would carry out tasks and which would pass them along. This led some inmates to only submit medical slips on certain shifts or direct them to specific members of staff. Janjak, a nurse in Men's Minimum, explained how he did not want other staff to see him doing specific tasks:

> My friend [fellow nurse] said, "Why are you taking this thing personally?" I said, "Because these are my patients". But I realised taking it personally I was making myself kind of notorious, you know. So, I listened to my

friend. And because there are a lot of things not getting done here, but I am not a supervisor. Because if I say something, it is going to become my job, you see.

5.2.3 Unequipped to Play Prison Games

Staff were unprepared to work in prison. Officer training contributed to a "tough guy" culture, leading some staff to actively degrade inmates. Degradation, in this case, was often done by young staff in order to show dominance over inmates. Young staff, as young as 18 years old, believed degradation helped establish a social position of authority. Officer White, an officer in Men's Maximum, reflected on her experience during a nine-week accreditation training course, explaining how it did little to prepare her for non-violent conflict resolution:

> [officer training] does not prepare you for walking in the facility and having an inmate come up to you. I could beat my face and do 400 sit-ups, and then the next day you put me in front of an inmate who's still going to be 400 pounds, bald, with "I hate niggers" tattooed across his eyebrows. That does not prepare me for that. How is you, as a drill sergeant yelling in my face, going to prepare me to deal with the white supremacists that I must come across when I walk in the door?

Dean, a training officer, developed and instructed the pre-service and in-service training for officers at Melville prison. He also inducted volunteers, healthcare workers, and other support staff. Dean recognised that the training course disproportionately focused on force. However, he said that his hands were tied when it came to teaching staff any alternative ways of managing inmate custody and control, explaining:

> We teach use of force. One of the things that we really do not cover enough on is understanding the inmate population. It is a very hard sell to sell to management and the union. But I'm going to tell you that of my 32 years plus being here, I have used more of my brain in communicating with inmates, and trying to understand where they're coming from, and that kind of thing, than I ever used a club, stick, baton, firearm, or pepper spray.

Empathy and the use of non-violent conflict resolution was more common among experienced officers, who acquired this disposition over time. Officer White, an officer in Men's Maximum, explained:

> You come across that with a veteran officer, somebody who's been around for 15-20 years, who has gained the respect of these inmates because these inmates have been in and out, their fathers have been in and out, their grandfathers have been in and out. You know, and a lot of new officers come in and they want to be big and bad, and they're like, "I got the badge", you know, "and I'm going to tell you what to do".

New officers were separated from veteran officers because of "bid to post" policy. Not surprisingly, "bid" staff often selected positions with limited inmate contact and in facilities with lower turnover. Thus, the staff who were least likely to degrade inmates and most likely to possess non-violent conflict resolution skills were removed from the frontlines. Officer Meeks, the medical dispensary officer in Men's Jail, thought that new staff should receive mentorship:

> I wish that [Melville] would tap into some of the older officers, including myself, to maybe address the Academy occasionally. This job is not for everybody. And do you know what? Other than the job itself, and what it takes to be this type of individual, if you're going to get – if you receive people differently, and you're going to be offended by all walks of life, all language of life, then this job isn't for you, because you can't let a gesture or a name bother you. Do you know what I mean? […] You must check your pride at the door.

The "bid to post" policy also restricted Brass from placing staff in roles best suited for their skills, such as posting empathetic staff to positions with greater inmate contact. Warden Cook, the warden of Women's Maximum, explained:

> The strength of the union here in [Melville] is amazing. It's nationally renowned. The fact that the officers have pick-up posts, where they can get into a bid, and they can work that bid indefinitely, unless you abolish the position, which means it limits the opportunity to offer people

different types of experiences. The fact that they pick the posts they work, and go to roll call and tell the shift commander where they're going to work each day, it's really crippling, and I think it thwarts the development of new officers.

This policy impacted the nursing staff who were in the same bargaining group as officers. "Bid to post" staff were stuck in the positions they had selected, which meant they would see the same inmate's day-in-and-day-out. Nursing staff, who dealt with inmate's complex health issues and the physical fallout of self-degradation, faced the real risk of internalising inmate's challenges. Warden Cook explained how she felt powerless to intervene when a staff member became exacerbated on the job:

In most institutional healthcare systems, people do consider the burnout factor. There are certain jobs that are more stressful than others. And under the [Union] provisions, you cannot exercise discretion in giving people a break. It's not like you can say "Do you know what? Go to Minimum for six months, catch your breath". It is like "Well, you've got that bid, you're stuck there".

5.2.4 Reduced Responsibility

Nurses were drawn, in part, to prison employment because it offered limited oversight and more autonomy. Despite nurses complaining about the workload in prison, they found the working conditions in the community to be even more difficult, as it required more bureaucratic paperwork and legal responsibility, like Gina, a nurse in Men's Jail, and Yolanda, a nurse in Women's Maximum, depicted:

Gina: So, when I got my license, I worked for [a community hospital], and that was atrocious, and I cried every day in the parking lot before I would go to work. I could not stand it. At your 41st hour, they would bring someone over and say they are taking over, and they would make you leave, you know. The documentation was gruelling. All you would do is fill out paperwork.

> *Yolanda*: I was burnt out in the nursing home. So, what happened is that I used to work from 3:00 to 11:00, and I would not get out, you know, until like 12:30 or 1:00 in the morning.

Linda, a nurse in Women's Maximum, also conveyed a similar sentiment to Gina and Yolanda, explaining that the physical labour in a community setting was too difficult and required too much responsibility:

> I was getting to an age where I knew hospital work was getting too much for me physically, I couldn't do it anymore, and they were cutting back on the nursing staff, and it was just getting to a point where it was brutal. It is for the young.

Nurses also worked overtime and reported equally taxing schedules in the prison, although the compensation for correctional nursing was far better than work in the community. Allen, a nurse in Men's Jail, described how the structure of the prison system typically allowed for frequent rests. It was not uncommon to see him napping in one of the clinical rooms throughout the duration of the study. He explained why this rest time was important for staff:

> See, because the [community] hospitals, we have a lot of critical care, and you got more overworked, you know, overload of work when you are working, and you don't get any help. Like I worked in the emergency room, and you are almost all the time on your feet. Hardly you take a break. You don't take an hour break, and you don't break the way we can break right here, because when there's a lockdown, there is not much to do, so we have time to catch up and rest.

I suspect that the disruption from a self-harming inmate when a nurse was resting was another factor contributing to the resentment staff expressed for playing prison games. Allen also described how prison nurses were less liable for negligence when compared to nurses in the community, explaining that "The job is totally different here. Like I say, we are nurses anywhere, but the job itself is much more different. Less liability than being in a regular hospital".

Healthcare staff was aware of the Estelle v. Gamble ruling, which defined prison medical care in terms of "deliberate indifference to serious medical needs". This ruling set a lower standard for the provision of medical care in prison when compared to the general public, whereby inmates were not protected from insufficient treatment stemming from an "accident, inadvertent behavior, or ordinary negligence" (Thompson, 2010, p. 638).

Nurses described how they were rarely terminated for misconduct. Dotty, a nurse in Men's Jail, explained how inmates would threaten to sue her, but the threats rarely prompted actions beyond an internal review, she explained:

> Often it is just a threat, it is stupid shit, and it never really makes the courts, even the court system that we have set up in here to get rid of frivolous claims. We enable them by giving them money just to shut them up, and that's wrong, but that's from the director [Prison Director]. When we have the lawyers calling the Medical Director, who will then call or put an e-mail to the doctor to say, "I have to see this guy because [...] and meanwhile I've got five slips because it's stupid. It's not anything".

Typically, healthcare delivery in a community setting was also be subject to external oversight from the Department of Health, ensuring that standards were being met and appropriate care delivered. However, it was also reported that the prison was a forgotten site when it came to surveillance from public health officials, as Janjack, a nurse in Men's Minimum, explained:

> The Department of Health doesn't breathe down your neck here. They don't really bother people here. [...] – like at a nursing home they will come at 5:00 a.m. If you do 11:00 to 7:00, they want to catch you in the act.

5.3 Creating Inmates as "Other"

Staff sought to distinguish themselves from inmates by discussing and displaying their wealth, which was most visible in community settings. Prison games became a site where staff punished inmates who they believed were undeserving or trying to gain benefits that were not earned. However, not all inmates were equally undeserving, and some inmates were seen as less deserving than others.

5.3.1 Performances of Wealth

I met Gina, a nurse in Men's Jail, at the Oakridge Supper Club. The scene was post-war Americana, and I imagined this was once a place where the white middle-class gathered to indulge in large Italian meals and cheap cocktails. Established in the 1930s, The Club was a single-story brick building tucked away in Melville's suburbs. It was a favourite dining spot for prison staff. "Something Stupid", a song by Frank Sinatra, billowed across the parking lot from a speaker above the main door. The restaurant was empty except for a few tough-looking men at the bar, and an elderly couple on the back patio. The decor was 1950s, with brown Naugahyde banquettes and fake oak panelled walls. Each table was neatly set with paper mats and a decorative candle. The vemue was not overly trendy but positioned close to the prison and catered to a local workforce. The patrons of this establishment knew each other and greeted one another as they arrived.

Gina entered The Club, she was dressed to the nines. Gesturing to her outfit, she laughed, and said "Hun, don't worry this isn't a date, I just like to *zhuzh* myself up on a night off". Ordering a bottle of wine, she knocked back a glass before we started to talk. Staff, like Gina, exhibited and discussed the wealth they gained from working at the prison:

> I'm putting away $13,600.00 [per year]. I think that is right, it's a good chunk of change. I have some wealth investment that I – you know, he's [financial investor] calling me. He wants me to give him another cheque or something, but it hasn't happened, because I worked like all last year,

> now that I've been working for the state, and I saved 20%, and I just bought another house.

The discussion and display of material wealth was part of conspicuous consumption. Veblen's theory of the leisure class indicates that individuals emulate consumption patterns of other persons situated at higher points in a social hierarchy (Veblen, 1899/2003). There are two ways wealth can be indicated; the performance of leisure activities and the lavish expenditure on goods and services. For staff, the accumulation of property indicated that they were productive members of society and had prowess in financial matters (Trigg, 2001, p. 99). Staff status derived from judgments that others in society made about their social position, and thus they felt the need to convincingly describe and display their wealth.

Throughout this study, staff described a range of leisure activities including, goat farming, travelling, and hunting exotic animals. They often brought up this information to demonstrate their accrued wealth in society. Staff also presented this conspicuous consumption in other ways. For example, officers regularly drove luxury trucks, kept them immaculately clean, and parked them across two or three parking spaces in the prison lot. Thus, families visiting inmates would need to park in an auxiliary lot and walk or take a bus to access the prison. This was done to showcase accumulated wealth to the visitors who often came from the same communities as staff.

For staff, showing wealth was more important than institutional symbols of distinction, such as an officer's uniform or badge. This presentation of a life associated with leisure transcended what they would typically have access to, if not for their employment in prison. More than this, staff sought to dissociate themselves from their occupation, as they believed that community members looked down on them as prison officers. Bourdieu, recognises such performances of wealth as relatively weak enactments of power and distinction, explaining "the naïve exhibitionism of 'conspicuous consumption', which seeks distinction in the crude display of ill-mastered luxury, is nothing compared to the unique capacity of a pure gaze, a quasi-creative power which sets the aesthetic apart from the common herd by a radical difference which seems to be inscribed in 'persons'" (Bourdieu, 1984/2010, p. 31). Thus, the presentation of wealth was a fragile display that staff did in order to show they were different from inmates.

5.3.2 Distinguishing Inmates as Undeserving

Some staff understood inmates game playing as an attempt to misuse the prison and state welfare system, recognising how this practice enabled inmates' access to benefits. Staff felt these benefits were generally underserved and recognised some inmates as less deserving than others. Staff believed prison was meant to be an institution of punishment. Therefore, additional punishment and suffering would need to be rendered when inmates were seen to be benefiting from this environment. Thus, staff policed prisoners' access to resources, documentation, and privileges to police moral and class boundaries. Linda, a nurse in Women's Maximum, expressed her disapproval and frustration at the level of treatment inmates could access in prison, a common sentiment among nursing staff:

> I'm very angry, extremely angry. The elderly can't afford to eat and buy medications. These are hard-working people that have worked all their lives. They have been law-abiding citizens. They have done everything they're supposed to do, and they get a kick in the ass when they get elderly [...] I've had to go and say I can't take that medication to the pharmacist, because it's $40.00 a month. And I come in here and see people that are getting $2,000.00 an injection. And I just think how obscene. You break the law, and you get treated better than the elderly in this country.

Staff depicted themselves as law-abiding citizens and hard-working Americans. They contrasted these perceptions with depictions of inmates as manipulative and "lazy", often failing to acknowledge the impossible challenges inmates might face in removing themselves from the criminal justice system. This perception sometimes included other groups of people that staff identified as undeserving, as Gina, a nurse in Men's Jail, explained:

> I know that laziness and entitlement is a choice. Do you know what? The rest of the world knows about these types of people, because if you don't work for something you can't possibly have pride. Now, I think some things can be done like border control to prevent the influx. I think we could do more in terms of immigration to make sure that we're not a dumping ground for everybody's sick, poor and needy, and that's what they know. They can take the Statue of Liberty and give it back to France, and I'll give you your sick, your poor, and we'll take care of my hairy buns. No, give it right back to France, get it out of Staten Island. Take it away. I'm sick of it.

Staff, exemplified by Gina, felt it was their moral duty to safeguard social and welfare resources from reaching inmates. They were acutely aware of their role, and the role of the prison, in enabling inmates' access to services. The staff felt the laws of society unfairly benefited inmates, as it provided a pathway to medical care, housing, and financial support. These were also the resources that staff did not obtain easily in their own lives, and were ironically achieved through "doing a bid" alongside inmates, as Gina explained:

> The government giveaways. I mean, really, honestly? Let me ask you a question. Why do I have to pass a piss test to earn a fucking paycheque, and you [inmates] don't have to pass any test to collect a welfare cheque? Why? I've got to pass a piss test to earn the job so I can work, so I can make money, so they can take my taxes and give it to you, and you can have every drug habit you want. The government's guilty; they are very guilty.

This resentment often turned into action when playing prison games. Allen, a nurse in Men's Minimum, described how staff viewed medical interventions for inmates as a complete waste of public resources. Staff recognised that health interventions had little effect in a system that did not rehabilitate offenders, as Allen explained:

> It is a waste in a way that these people are not rehabilitated whatsoever. The Methadone [opioid replacement therapy] is supposed to be for someone like you and me. Let us say you have an addiction, and you are a healthy worker, hard-working person, you have something to go in front of you for your life. Most of these guys, they have no jobs. They are just addicted to the Methadone, and that is all it is. Enough of these people have no jobs. That is what I think is a waste.

This sentiment played out in the decisions staff made when providing or withholding medical care to inmates. Punishment was often rendered to those understood to be less deserving than others. Brian, a nurse in Men's Medium, recounted his interaction with an inmate during a clinical consultation. His account demonstrates how some nursing staff reflected on an inmate's criminal record when making healthcare decisions:

> So, I kind of reminded him, "Do you know what? You need to pay for this". "Why should I? You owe it". "No, I don't owe you anything. You owe your victims, so in fact that I think you should pay for every little thing you can while you're in here as partial payment to your victims". And of course, if I'd kept it going, we would have an argument, you know.

According to staff, some inmates were less deserving of rehabilitation and care when compared to other inmates. Staff made this determination through an inmate's criminal conviction, and if they could relate to the inmate's crime. Tanya, an inmate in Women's Maximum, was an inmate staff considered to be particularly undeserving of care. She was a former healthcare worker, now serving a 40-year sentence for strangling her child. Her crime was frequently publicised in the news, depicting how she strangled her young child and placed her lifeless body into bed, pulling up the covers and tucking her in for the night. After committing this crime, Tanya attempted to take her own life.

Tanya was enrolled in my "Butts & Guts" exercise class, which I ran twice-weekly in Women's Maximum. We built a rapport in-between star jumps and push-ups. Tanya was targeted by staff because of her crime, and described how she was often verbally berated, had her privileges restricted, and received excessive punishment for minor infractions. Staff were not subtle in their punishment towards Tanya, for example, I overheard one officer on the second-floor landing yell, “Hey Tanya, you fucking killed your child. How does it feel to be a fucking child killer? Go to hell”.

Tanya was an inmate that the staff could relate to; she previously worked in a profession that was considered core to the prison operation. As such, her biography was something that enabled them to see themselves in the offender population. Further, she committed a crime involving a minor, which staff saw as morally objectionable.

Further to this, and much like the “little shock bombs” used during staff communication, exemplified by Warden Cook earlier in this Chapter, it was through staff members visible chastisement of an inmate that staff signalled to colleagues where their moral boundaries lie. Officer White, an officer in Men’s Maximum, also depicted how she singled out inmates and what type of degradation she might inflict on these individuals:

Officer White: Because there’s respect. I can have more respect for a person who robbed a bank to feed their family than for somebody who had sex with their granddaughter. [...] “Okay, so you stabbed your wife 30 times”. “She was in bed with somebody. My heart was broken, I was hurt by it”. Hey, do you know what? I would probably do the same thing.

Landon: So, do certain inmates get treated differently in prison?

Officer White: Absolutely. By inmate society and officer society, they are completely shunned, completely, absolutely.

Landon: What kind of things happen to them?

Officer White: They get treated awful. Pretty much they just get treated like they are dogs, like they are trash.

Landon: What specifically?

Officer White: It is more tone, disgust, and you have that in your conversations, you know. I had a guy one time who had sex with an 18-month-old baby, broke her hips, broke her legs just to penetrate, and once I knew that’s what he had done—you know, he was a very needy inmate, he always needed something. “Can I do this, can I do that, can I do this?” And to anybody else, it would be like, “Yeah, sure,

> go back up to your room, go grab your coat, you know, I'll let you in". But to him "No, we're not letting you in". "But I need my coat". "You should have grabbed it, sorry", you know. "But why?" "Why? Well, I don't know. Why did you rape an 18-month-old baby?"

Officer White also offered a reflection as to why this inmate's crime was so relatable and led her to treat him differently, explaining, "You know, I think about my own children, and I am just disgusted, absolutely disgusted".

A moral code was not something exclusively held up by the staff in prison, rather inmates also depicted a hierarchy of who was more or less deserving of respect. Freddie, an inmate in Men's Maximum, illustrated this pecking order during a discussion:

> Ok, so at the bottom of the hierarchy, you have got your child diddlers [child sex offenders]. They are at the total bottom. They kind of stay out of sight and out of mind and form their own little group. Above paedophiles would be your little rapers and domestic guys - guys who got to beat up on the old lady. Then after that, you've got your lifers… there are some lifers who get a higher respect like [inmates name] - like the man has been here since back in the day… he started his bid in 1973. He is well respected and was connected at one time. Then you have got some lifers like the guy who killed his mother and father and buried them out back in the septic tank […]

This chapter has outlined the cultural milieu of prison staff by highlighting structural and social factors that underpin their positions in prison games. Staff and inmates have similar biographical experiences in both the community and in prison. Their social circles often overlap, and boundaries are crossed. Inmates and staff both rely on the prison as a site of capital, enabling them to ascend social positions traditionally outside their grasp. These conditions create a fragile distinction between members of staff and the offending population, leading some staff to police social and moral boundaries through actively degrading inmates.

The next chapter will continue to explore prison games from the perspective of the staff. This chapter will examine how staff become enculturated into a system of punishment over time. It will explore the consequences of some staff who feel like they do not matter in their professional work. This chapter will also examine how staff often become restricted from providing care in the prison setting, and how some staff might resist these imposed constraints.

References

Bourdieu, P. (1984/2010). *Distinction: A social critique of the judgement of taste.* London: Routledge (Reprint 2010).

National Center for Educational Statistics. (2014). *The condition of education 2014 (NCES 2014-083), annual earnings of young adults.* U.S. Department of Education: Washington, D.C. Retrieved from http://nces.ed.gov/fastfacts/display.asp?id=77.

Thompson, J. H. (2010). Today's deliberate indifference: Providing attention without providing treatment to prisoners with serious medical needs. *Harvard Civil Rights-Civil Liberties Law Review, 45*(2), 635–654.

Trigg, A. B. (2001). Veblen, Bourdieu, and conspicuous consumption. *Journal of Economic Issues, XXXV*(1), 99–115.

Veblen, T. (1899/2003). *The theory of the leisure class a Penn state electronic classic series publication.* Retrieved from http://www.wilsonsd.org/cms/lib01/PA01000270/Centricity/Domain/185/Theory-Leisure-Class.pdf.

6

From Care to Corrections

6.1 The System Changes You

In the beginning, officers viewed their prison employment as a stepping-stone for loftier public service ambitions. Nurses depicted how they entered the field of corrections to provide care to people with complex health needs. However, over time their understanding of prison changed, and staff described being drawn into a world of punishment.

For officers, the prison was an opportunity to change their social positions. At the time of this research, prison officers expressed wanting to be community police officers, viewing this profession as a more prestigious and respected position. Dean, a training officer, explained:

> A lot of the folks, a lot of the agencies out there have recognised us as a good stepping-stone to State Police: there are probably 10 of my graduates that are State troopers. As a matter of fact, the colonel of the State Police was a correctional officer. He was one of my graduates. Fire Departments take from here. Most PDs [police departments] take guys from here. If you have got a good record, you will do okay.

L. Kuester, *Violence in Pursuit of Health*, Palgrave Studies in Prisons and Penology, https://doi.org/10.1007/978-3-030-61350-1_6

Many officers never transitioned from correctional officer to community police, often explaining that a good salary and pension kept them in the field of corrections. However, their desire to join a community police force is telling for what it reveals about their motivations for becoming an officer, as well as how their initial hopes were undermined by the prison regime, as Pep, a retired prison officer, explained:

> I think years ago, I had a very different perspective of what Corrections was about. I wanted to be in law enforcement. My goal was to do a few years here and go on to like the [State Police] and be a State police officer. And at 20 years old, I was very naive to the fact that – I thought public service was public service. [...] And when I first started working in Corrections, I found that it was more punitive. The job was to catch people doing things wrong.

Staff found it challenging to embrace a system of punishment, depicting how their duties in prison, at least for some, led them to withdraw from interacting with inmates, express apathy towards providing care, and generally accept that active degradation was a part of the job. Nurses described developing a "correctional officer mentality" over time, as Gina, a Nurse in Men's Jail, described:

> The same way to ask why did you become a correctional officer and you're not a nurse anymore, knowing that you don't have no sympathy, no compassion for the patients you're dealing with? The same way with everybody, because that's what changes. [...] I think that a lot of them [correctional officers] are so brutal, nasty and everything. So why did you change? Are you the same way at home?

Several nurses described having a dual role as both a prison officer and a nurse. This group of healthcare staff found it necessary to adopt social characteristics from each position. However, generally, when nursing staff depicted adopting a "correctional officer mentality" they were embracing a punishment regime. Nurses sought to balance the delivery of care and the provision of punishment, as Nina and Linda, both nurses in Women's Maximum, explained:

Linda: Both [correctional officer and nurse]—we are Correctional Officer Hospital II […] You've got to be firm. When you are working with inmates, you have got to be firm, because you are working with a whole different animal.

Nina: But there's a degree of nurses I think that fall into the correction officer mode because it's strict and structured, and they tend to—I don't want to say lose their compassion, but they tend to mimic the officers, and are a little more rigid than I would expect.

Nurses found it necessary to adopt a harsh stance when interacting with inmates. This was critical to playing prison games, which, according to nurses, required them to restrict inmates' access to certain treatments and benefits. Reggie, a nurse in Men's Jail, explained how she would take on a correctional officer persona when assessing inmates during sick call, saying "Oh, they [inmates] know me. They wouldn't dare try and play me".

Nurses did not enter their prison careers by wanting to become an officer. Instead, many nurses expressed that they were initially motivated, in part, to work in a prison setting because they would be supporting the rehabilitation of offenders by improving their health. However, Reggie, like her colleagues, depicted how adopting an officer mentality made it exceptionally difficult to return to the role of care. She explained how she, and many of her co-workers, were no longer able to work in settings where a higher level of care was required:

> A lot of us say if we ever had to go back on a floor in a hospital, you would probably be fired within two nights. We would because we have -- even now. We have a mentality now when you are here that long, you are used to saying "No" and "Go". It is my way or the highway. "No, you're not getting that". Or "Get out of my face, I'm not dealing with you". I could never go back, you know, because I know what is in the hospital ---

Yolanda, a nurse in Women's Maximum, described how playing prison games limited nurse's future employment prospects. She believed playing prison games turned her into a certain type of nurse, a nurse who "lacked humanity". Yolanda highlighted how prison nurses operate under different social rules when compared to nurses in the community, which led to feelings of isolation within the profession:

> Basically, it's going to be hard for me to go to the hospital now, or to go to a nursing home, because I have to retrain myself, because I have that mentality already, like I have to be guarded every time, so [...] It is hard, yeah, yeah. They [inmates] know what you can think, and they know what they can get over you. They know that. They know whom they can manipulate easily.

There was evidence of healthcare staff being inducted into a correctional officer mentality upon taking up prison employment. Though, I suspect it was more common for new staff to discreetly adopt a punitive stance over time by becoming caught up in the workforce culture, which was a space averse to showing weakness and compassion, as Warden Cook depicted in Chapter 5. However, an officer mentality was endorsed among staff arriving in the prison, as John, a nurse in Men's Minimum, described:

> [...] when the new nurses come in, you can see other nurses, or even correctional staff, "Hey, this is how we do it here. A guy comes up...". So, they try to influence them. I have seen guys come and go. "Hey, you're back in. What did you do this time?" Do you know what I mean? I don't like say "I'm all set with you; I'm all done with you. I'm not going to help you because you've come in and out many times". But especially the new nursing staff, I have seen some of the older nurses, and the correctional staff we have mentioned, try to influence the way -- how they would treat them [inmates].

Taken together, the staff in prison embodied a punishment regime that isolated them from mainstream society. Over time, staff did not fit in with the job they set off to do, nor the aspirations they set off to achieve. In the context of imprisonment, punishment was infectious and dominated how staff came to see their professional role and responsibility over time.

6.2 Not Mattering

For a person to "matter", they must have the capacity to make a difference in the world around them (Elliott, Kao, & Grant, 2004). Mattering in what you do is important for your idea of self, and how you see yourself contributing to society (Rosenberg & McCullough, 1981). The feeling of not mattering can lead to low self-esteem and depression (Rosenberg & McCullough, 1981; Taylor & Turner, 2001) and limit a person's ability to deliver care (Pearlin & LeBlanc, 2001).

Staff described not mattering in their professional work. This arose from feeling complicit in a punishment system that did not discourage crime, nor did it effectively rehabilitate offenders. Prison work was hard, and despite adopting an officer mentality, many staff wanted better psychological support. When inmates played prison games, nurses understood these actions to undermine their delivery of care and rehabilitation. Officers perceived prison games to weaken their ability to maintain control over the institution. Collectively, the staff felt powerless to effect positive change in the context of imprisonment.

While most staff preferred to receive positive attention, failing this, staff would act in a socially undesirable way, as it would mean not being ignored; negative attention was better than no attention at all, as Dr. McGreevy, an HIV consultant to the prison, explained:

> And if you are a nurse or correctional officer, when you do something helpful for someone, you matter, but also, when you manipulate the system to provoke a person, or cause them pain, you know, or dig at them, however you want to call it, you also matter, you are somebody. And society does not only treat inmates as if they don't matter, but they also treat correctional officers a little bit like they don't matter […]

6.2.1 Staff Were Complicit in a Failed System

Complicity in a "failed system" happened when staff perceived their professional work to have little to no positive effect. Staff was required to participate in a system that perpetuated prison games by mandating they deliver punishment, even while recognising that an inmate's violation was done to capitalise on a predicted penalty.

When inmates self-degraded or did not follow medical advice, nurses felt their efforts were undercut, and thus, over time, withheld care. For example, Linda, a nurse in Women's Maximum, described how she refused care to an inmate who was not following a medical intervention:

> She threw it away in the trash, and then said she wanted another one upon her next bid here. And I wanted to say, "You're not going to order that again; are you?" And I have fought with the doctors and made enemies. I have been very verbal about it.

Officers found it emotionally challenging to punish inmates for playing prison games. This regularly led them to become exacerbated, as they recognised there was no way to end a cycle of punishment connected to rights and benefits for inmates. Officer Lazzeri, an officer in Women's Maximum, described how it was difficult not to be frustrated, explaining:

> I know what I am capable of. And as human as you are, and as empathetic as you want to be, you get pushed and tested, and I just – I do not want to become a rotten person. And then they badger and badger, and then you go to a side of yourself, for me, that I am not proud or happy to be that person.

Staff worked under a prison regime that was not always humane or just but nevertheless required punishment, such as placing an inmate in segregation. The staff did not necessarily see punishments as effective but rather mandated by the institution's policy and practice. Officer Lazzeri depicted how it was upsetting to regularly put inmates in segregation, particularly for extended periods:

> Whatever she did, she still a human being. I mean, you would not want a skunk to be living in a little cell like that for a year, for real. We do not like the smell of skunks, but I think each and every one of us would feel sorry for that skunk after a while, even if it sprayed us. Are we going to want to hurt it? No, we probably want to let it out after a while. I mean, a year, that is excessive.

At the time of this study, Samantha, the deputy director of Rehabilitation Services, was retiring from a 33-year career in the prison service. She was an artist and started her career by coordinating Melville's offender arts programme. Samantha served as the warden of Women's Maximum for ten years, before becoming an administrator. She depicted how staff, at all levels, were required to suppress their discontent with a heavy-handed punishment regime:

> And what about people who have mental illness, who end up in segregation cells 23 hours a day for 10 years in a row? Look at High Security. We have got guys buried in High Security. And that is with well-meaning people. Yeah, you know, you are catching me at a time when I am about -- I am okay now acknowledging my disgust, and it is something that I have had to suppress. In order to survive here, I've had to compromise around those issues that would have driven me out of the system.

6.2.2 An Impossible Mission

Melville prison's mission statement calls for the institution to deter crime, punish offenders through restricting their freedom, and rehabilitate offenders to become productive, law-abiding citizens. In many respects, these were impractical tasks for staff to achieve under a system of prison games. Not meeting institutional objectives, or even coming close to meeting them, led staff to feel their work did not matter, or at least did not matter in a positive way.

Imprisonment restricted offenders' freedom, rendered punishment, and delivered a range of rehabilitation services, including medical and public healthcare, addiction support, mental health, anger management, education, vocational training, and arts programming. However, the prison largely did not "rehabilitate offenders", nor did it deter crime.

In 2014, 50% of offenders returned to prison within 3-years of their release. This included 37% of female offenders and 52% of male offenders, who, on average, only spent 11-months in the community before being reincarcerated. While long-term data is not available for the research site, a U.S. Department of Justice report indicates that the recidivism rate increases significantly over time. This study found that

86% of state prisoners released in 2005, across 30 states, were rearrested at least once during the 9-year follow-up period (Alper, Dorose, & Markman, 2018).

While the prison was a place where offenders were punished by losing their freedom, it was also a site where, through prison games, they gained a pathway to benefits that were difficult to attain elsewhere in the community. Prison offered people the right to healthcare, shelter, and food, or as Pep, a retired prison officer explained, "for violating somebody's rights, whether it is your own rights or another's, you actually gain rights for coming to prison".

Staff recognised the impossible challenge of delivering rehabilitation within a context of prison games, like Allen, a nurse in Men's Minimum, and Linda, a nurse in Women's Maximum, exemplified:

Allen: You leave today, and then you come back a month later. So, I do not know what the deterrent is.
Linda: It is not rehabilitating. We are housing them here. We are not teaching them a thing. We are not doing anything for them. We are just not teaching them skills to live on the outside. I would fail, I would fail.

The staff made connections to laws and politics that underpinned offenders' regular return to prison, which undermined the rehabilitative component of their jobs. Many staff understood their role was to, however perversely, deliver social welfare services to offenders who struggled to access in the community, as Gina a nurse in Men's Jail and Linda, a nurse in Women's Maximum, explained:

Gina: Most of these guys, I do not think you can rehabilitate, because there is a lot of factors. How can you rehabilitate somebody who's 90 years old, coming in from a nursing home that was a dump. Can you rehabilitate a 35-year-old junkie? He ain't never getting out. He's not getting off the stuff. You know, you are not going to rehabilitate them.
Linda: These girls are destined to fail; I hate to say it. I look at them and think we are not doing a thing. We are spending so much money housing these women for what? For what? For nothing. I am frustrated, I am frustrated. I get angry. I tell people. I open my mouth, I cause problems, I get in trouble, and then, you know, it is just—it is just a

> circle. They are going to come back. You know they are going to be back. If not, they are going to die.

Observing a high recidivism rate led some staff to feel as though nothing they did would matter, and as a result, staff withheld care to try and remove themselves from a system that they perceived wasn't working in a positive way, as Dotty, a Nurse in Men's Jail, depicted:

> Because they come back. Some of them come back two weeks later, and they are back on all the shit [drugs] that they got off. And it is like sometimes why do we bother?

6.2.3 Experience of Shame

Staff, like inmates, experienced stigma from their association to the prison. This led staff to refuse to talk about their work to others, as well as hide institutional symbols upon leaving the prison. Staff worried about the public perception of prison officers and believed others thought of them as "thugs" and "underachieving". Officer Rodgers, an officer in Women's Maximum, and Dean, a prison training officer, explained the public perception of prison officers in this way:

> *Officer Rodgers*: "People think we are dumb, that we're uneducated, or we're wannabe cops, or we stay here because we couldn't be a cop".
>
> *Dean*: So, yeah, I think the perception is—I think society's perception of the—and the media does not do a good job of portraying us. When you look at Shawshank Redemption, I do not think they showed a legit correctional officer. Every correctional officer is either mean or is beating on somebody. Sort of, you know, we are portrayed very poorly.

Nurses and officers were reluctant to talk about their work to others outside the prison, which included concealing aspects of their work from close family and friends. Staff feared that they would be judged negatively by the work they did, which often contributed to feelings of isolation, as Reggie, a nurse in Men's Jail, depicted:

> Because they ask too many questions, and I do not want to talk about it. I cannot because people are just blown away [...] they would not understand. If you said that, if you said that they smear shit, they would have -- most people would not even think of that. And what I am amazed is that a lot of people do it.

Staff engaged in another ritual, which was to disguise their profession from the public by removing institutional symbols before entering and upon exiting the prison. This included taking off their uniform and removing their identity badge. In some cases, this was done for safety, as staff and inmates often came from the same community, and thus there was concern they would be recognised by a disgruntled ex-inmate or someone that, because of their uniform, might wish to do them harm. However, a lot of the time, this ritual was because staff felt stigmatised by the public, as Officer White, an officer in Men's Maximum, described:

> So even if you are a good officer, you still get a little chip, because you know you are going to get treated differently. I've had people tell me, "Make sure when you go to the supermarket to take off your uniform first, because you'll get treated differently" [...] Nine times out of 10 you have a male officer, he will change his uniform because he doesn't want anybody to know where he works. Because it takes one officer to make us all look bad, and the news blows it up; do you know what I mean? And it could be something stupid, you know, officer got caught with some weed [marijuana]. So what? Big deal, you know.

6.2.4 A Lack of Support

The staff did not feel supported by the prison system. According to front-line staff, the Brass did not ask for their opinions, insight, and thoughts about how the prison should operate. More than this, the staff reported a lack of praise when they did something above and beyond their duty. Staff depicted how their complaints were often slow-walked or failed to arise to the attention of administrators. Officer Rodgers, an officer in

Women's Maximum, exemplified how staff felt overlooked in the prison setting:

> Yeah, it's not a glamorous job, and you're in here all the time, and everything's always with an order, always telling you what to do, and you may have more experience in something, and it really doesn't matter what you think in here. Your opinions do not mean shit in this place, and that's a pretty strangulated environment to be in for someone who -- me, I'm hands-on, I'm a thinker. I am always problem-solving.

Some staff shared with me their ideas about improving relationships between themselves and inmates. However, the staff also expressed a reluctance to bring their ideas to prison administrators, believing the administration could not implement them because of institutional rules. This was exemplified by Officer Lazzeri, an officer in Women's Maximum, when she described an idea for a public health intervention:

> Right, because I cannot get personal with anyone as officer to inmate, because then I've crossed a boundary. And it is a shame, because there's a lot that could be shared. I can give advice, you know, I can tell you [inmate] to wash your hands, I can tell you are coughing terrible.

When staff went beyond their duty, which might include working unpaid overtime, comforting an inmate in segregation, or volunteering to take on extra tasks, their actions went without appropriate praise and endorsement from senior staff, as Officer Rodgers, an officer in Women's Maximum, explained:

> I have stayed late because I -- like it has happened a few times. I used to go down to ISO [segregation unit] and try to talk to them when they were about to like form a team [tactical response team] to go in at them, and I come in and like, you know, "Come on, you do this". And without wanting to work overtime, I've kind of -- do you know what? I will just keep -- because I've kind of built a rapport with the inmate, I will just go to the emergency room with them, you know. And then something will happen where it is like -- you know, like they act like I never done anything. I do not know, it is just like forget about that.

Certain grievances were seen to be slow-walked by the administration. When this happened, staff described playing their own prison games with Brass, by playing up a complaint or filing a false grievance. For example, Janjak, a nurse in Men's Minimum, described using his race to resolve a dispute he was having with a deputy warden. According to Janjak, he would racialise his complaints to draw the attention of administrators, he explained:

> They are afraid. They do not want to be called racist, but it is there in their head. So the only reason they're not doing that, they know you have an open mouth, they know you are bold, when you do that they want you -- when they do that to me, I will understand, and I will use the word on them that they don't want to hear. I use it. I will tell them -- like the deputy, I told him he was a colonial master. Yeah, I called him that. I said, "You're a colonial master waiting for a slave to be guillotined". I wrote six pages, and I called him all the names that could be applied to a situation like that, and he wept.

Staff also conveyed a need for better psychological support because of their job. Samantha, the deputy director of Rehabilitation Services, reflected on the mental challenge of prison work:

> I will not be sorry to say goodbye to all these thoughts, really, because, you know, ten years of living with those inmates, it was hard. It is very sad. You know, it is a lot of loss, and a lot of failure. Most people do not have that much loss and failure in their lives, or even know that. It's not like I was living it personally, but I knew about it every day, and it takes its toll on you.

Throughout this study, I built close relationships with participants during interviews and through ethnographic immersion. There was an unavoidable therapeutic element to these encounters, both for the participants and for me as a researcher. Our conversations highlighted a need for staff to receive better psychological support. For example, this is how Officer Lazzeri, an officer in Women's Maximum, viewed our private conversations:

Officer Lazzeri: Sometimes, we are just dying for an outlet. Maybe that's why people talk to you as much and as long as they do, because it's a sense of calm, and our insides are uptight. We could be here, and then the next minute I am going to a Code Blue, and what do I do? I go out there and someone is hanging, their eyes are rolled behind their head, or someone is cut the crap out of themselves, they are bleeding, freaking out, you know. So, I mean, it is that, and you do not have anywhere to go with that.

Officer Lazzeri: Well, you know, I took the girl right down. It was traumatising for me. Nobody ever asked me about how I felt that day. Yeah, Then I found out like three weeks later they were going to write me up, because they were worried about a lawsuit against them, and because they had these rules that were implemented that were not good.

6.2.5 Institutional Barriers to Care

On a typical Thursday afternoon, I would put on my gym kit and walk to the Women's Minimum visitation centre. The space would be repurposed into a gym for my "Butts and Guts" class, a twice-weekly exercise class that rotated through the prison facilities. The women would move the long tables and wooden benches to the side of the room plug in a boombox, and do 45 minutes of exercise. The class was not just about physical training but offered a space where inmates could socialise, laugh, and sing to music. This was a space of enjoyment, for both me and the inmates.

However, even in this space of relative enjoyment, there were regular reminders of how difficult it was to show care or even physical contact in prison. Cameras monitored each exercise class. On occasion, an exercise would crossed the line and draw attention from the substation's security staff. For example, this included holding an inmate's ankles while doing leg raises or wheelbarrowing each other across the room. When this happened, an officer would appear at the door and say, "No touching, touching is forbidden". There was also a large sign listing the rules that visitors were required to follow when meeting inmates. This included no kissing, no long embraces, only embraces of short duration at the beginning and end of a visit, hands always above the table, and no loud and abrasive language. While serving an important security function, all these rules created an environment that physically and socially separated people.

Prison policies, particularly disciplinary practices, restricted the ability to display care. Staff often focused on small things, such as controlling objects, touching, language, expression of emotion, with the idea that regulating minor infractions would prevent larger transgressions, such as a riot. However, this created a heavily policed environment. Freddie, and inmate in Men's Maximum, depicted how it felt to go without feeling cared for over an extended period of time:

> It is more of a caring thing. It is really funny that as human beings, there comes a time when you have been incarcerated so long that you need to find someone to love. Everyone just wants to be loved, and everyone wants to love somebody.

Solitary confinement was another example of a disciplinary practice that resulted in staff becoming restricted from showing care. In Melville, all facilities, except for Minimum, held inmates in solitary confinement. Under these conditions, inmates were restricted from human contact, access to exercise, sunlight, and other forms of stimulation. Prison records suggest that up to 23% of the inmate population lived under conditions of solitary confinement, many of whom were designated as having a severe and persistent mental illness.

Segregation cells limit human contact and sensory experience. Thus, confinement involved housing an inmate in a small cell, typically 6-by-8 feet, for 22 to 24-hours a day. In this space, an inmate would sleep, eat, and use the toilet. Inmates would live like this for weeks, months, and sometimes years. Each segregation cell had a "trap" where food and medication would be delivered, and a small observation window looking on to the corridor. The cells had limited furniture, sometimes only a bed and toilet, and each room was monitored by a camera. Typically, an inmate was only let out of the cell to go to a "rec pen" for one hour a day or shower three times per week. Inmates reported not having access to basic amenities such as toilet paper and medication under these conditions.

There is well-documented evidence that solitary confinement negatively impacts a person's mental health, causing anxiety, panic, withdrawal, hallucinations, self-mutilation, and suicidal thoughts and behaviours (Grassin, 2006). Further, data from this study suggests that placing inmates in solitary confinement was distressing for the staff who inflicted this consequence. Staff were regularly required to deliver this inhumane punishment to offenders. While trauma experienced by inmates should not be minimised, it is also important to recognise that staff also struggled to reconcile this level of punishment. This was exemplified by Officer Lazzeri and Samantha earlier in this Chapter, who both described their disgust and emotional anguish with having to participate in, and bear witness to, this punishment.

This was why, in part, staff adopted an unempathetic stance towards inmates. Staff needed to see inmates as less than human, or at least less like themselves, to deliver this punishment. Restricting care enabled staff a degree of dehumanisation and psychological separation from the offender population.

The punishment regime, ranging from minor rules restricting contact to solitary confinement, underpinned a social culture that repressed care. Any demonstration of care and compassion by staff was seen as going against an underlying culture of punishment. Thus, providing care was socially policed. For example, Alan, a nurse in Men's Minimum, described receiving push-back from colleagues when displaying respect to inmates:

> If you helped an inmate out, some correctional officers would give you an attitude. So that component was the toughest thing I had to adjust to. It was not really my nursing skills, what I would do when I had a patient in front of me, and my assessment skills. It was sometimes after I dealt with a patient, they would leave, and the officer would say, "Do you know that guy? He killed someone", or "He's a child molester, and how can you take care of him?" That kind of thing. So that was the biggest

thing, dealing with security, and how they would try to influence what I would do with the patient.

A culture of punishment was not only enforced by officers but rather was quintessential to the prison environment. The treatment of inmates went beyond withholding care, and often included limiting anything understood to be humanising. The staff who humanised inmates were branded "giveaways", as Officer Lazzeri, an officer in Women's Maximum, and Dean, a training officer, described:

Officer Lazzeri: And they call you a giveaway if you are an officer and you work out there, and you try to look out for the inmate. You see that they have like mental health issues. Do you know what? I sent her home with a clean pair of underwear. The lady had no underwear. Her bra was as brown as that mailbox. Obviously, she had nothing. [...] Why wouldn't I give her a pair? She has no underwear. This is a woman. You know, how is she going to have any dignity? She is shaking, and you can tell she's not playing with a full deck, but at least she has a brand-new pair of underwear now.

Dean: My first couple of years on the job, because I gave inmates a toothbrush—you know, the toothbrush they should have had, blankets, towels, sheets, they branded me an inmate lover.

Displaying care towards inmates was also seen as a sign of weakness and vulnerability when it came to staff playing prison games, as Gina, a nurse in Men's Jail, described:

Yes, there would be, yes, yes, because other people will look at that as you befriended them, or the inmate thinks that you're their friend, and they can -- then they can begin to coerce you and manipulate you, which they're all expert at. So, it is a safety thing, and they [officers] do not want us brought into that.

Some staff resisted the punishment regime in often subtle ways. For example, Ritchie, a nurse in Men's Supermax, described how he would open communication lines with inmates residing in solitary confinement. Under these conditions, inmates would communicate with one another by yelling into the ventilation system or yelling loud enough so that others could hear them through the walls. Ritchie used the same communication method when delivering medications. He did this to demonstrate to inmates that he was there to help and, if needed, he would be willing to provide them care and support at the medical dispensary, Ritchie explained:

> Right. So, I do things regularly to build little bridges of communication. An example would be last week one of the guys had an appointment for a procedure. He was anxious about it because it had to happen relatively soon. But I knew the date. But I went down into the mod [housing unit] just to let him -- when the mod was quiet, but they can all hear. So I said to him, well aware that the whole mod could hear me, I said, "Hey, it's going to happen this week, very soon. Are you okay?" Now, I did that for him, to lower his anxiety, but I also had everybody listening to me.

I also participated in small acts of resistance against the punishment regime when it came to shackling practices during interviews. When interviewing inmates in solitary confinement, I always requested that the escorting officer uncuff the inmate or re-cuff them so that their arms were in front of their body. I did this knowing the requests would often be denied. However, this was done to show that I wanted the participant to be comfortable during an interview, signalling my desire for trust and care.

This chapter highlights the structural and social conditions that created a culture of punishment for staff. It describes how staff did not start off wanting to be punishers but became enculturated into this role over time through structuring mechanisms. Staff worked in a system that was understood to be failing in the rehabilitation of offenders. Taken together, these conditions led some staff to feel like they did not matter in their work, or at least matter positively. For staff to carry out a punishment regime, they needed to dehumanise inmates, explaining why some staff members' actively degraded this group of people.

The book's discussion will draw together a theory of prison games, as brought to light through different types of degradation between staff and inmates. It will look to other national models of imprisonment for contextualisation and comparison, offering a starting point for how

America might take steps towards reforming the experiences of offenders living with HIV and the prison staff who oversee them.

References

Alper, M., Dorose, M. R., & Markman, J. (2018). *2018 update on prisoner recidivism: A 9-Year follow-up period (2005–2014).* U.S. Bureau of Justice Statistics: Washington, DC. Retrieved from https://www.bjs.gov/index.cfm?ty=pbdetail&iid=6266.

Elliott, G. C., Kao, S., & Grant, A. (2004). Mattering: Empirical validation of a social-psychological concept. *Self and Identity, 3*, 339–354.

Grassin, S. (2006). Psychiatric effects of solitary confinement. *Washington University Journal of Law & Policy, 22*. Retrieved from https://openscholarship.wustl.edu/cgi/viewcontent.cgi?article=1362&context=law_journal_law_policy.

Pearlin, L. I., & LeBlanc, A. J. (2001). Bereavement and the Loss of Mattering. In T. J. Owens, S. Stryker & N. Goodman (Eds.), *Extending self-esteem theory and research* (pp. 285–300). New York, NY: Cambridge University Press.

Rosenberg, M., & McCullough, B. C. (1981). Mattering: Inferred significance and mental health. *Research in community and mental health, 2*(163–182).

Taylor, J., & Turner, R. J. (2001). A longitudinal study of the role and significance of mattering to others for depressive symptoms. *J Health Soc Behav, 42*(3), 310–325.

Discussion: Degradation and Prison Games

Degradation, expressed through the social process of prison games, was a key finding from a study that set out to explore the lived experience of inmates living with HIV. These concepts offer a theory of how violence was reproduced through imprisonment and connected to a benefits marketplace for health and welfare. Within this marketplace, degradation was used as a type of capital for both inmates and staff. Inmates often sought access to rights and resources otherwise difficult to obtain in the community, while staff used degradation to police inmates' social positions and deliver punishment. Prison games required participants to produce and use a range of *abjectionable*, illicit, and uncitizenly behaviour that perpetuated dependence on the prison system. Degradation included overt acts (e.g., swallowing razor blades) and subtle actions (e.g., talking back) that were quintessential to the prison environment. Prison games were played between people, as well as against the structuring mechanisms of the prison. On the one hand, prison games were a practice imbued with agency. On the other hand, it stripped agency by requiring participant's engage in debasement, physical harm, and returns to the prison over time.

Research findings are presented across four empirical chapters, drawing on accounts from inmates and staff. Chapter 3 introduces

L. Kuester, *Violence in Pursuit of Health*, Palgrave Studies in Prisons and Penology, https://doi.org/10.1007/978-3-030-61350-1

concepts of degradation and prison games at the site of healthcare. This chapter depicts three types of degradation in prison: self-degradation, degradation by others, and structural degradation. Degradation of the self involved inmate's use of their body, objects, or social positions, escalateing over time from small acts of debasement to extreme self-harming behaviour. Inmates degraded themselves to demonstrate a severe medical need that would gain attention from staff. Degradation by others, or active degradation, involved staff degrading inmates to police social and moral boundaries and deliver punishment. For staff, this included denying or delaying care to inmates, requiring performances of illness, and verbal debasement. Structuring mechanisms of the prison enabled prison games, which included, but were not limited to, legislation directing the type of healthcare inmates receive, internal grievance procedures and external litigation, as well as a punishment regime with predictable consequences for any transgression. No one was exempt from playing prison games, despite that inmates and staff understood the process differently through their own *habitus*. Staff and inmates both entered the field of imprisonment, where capital was won and lost through the playing of prison games.

Chapter 4 explores the benefits of prison games for inmates. This chapter outlines how staff and inmates might understand the playing of prison games differently, thus providing an initial understanding of how the two groups might justify their engagement in this social practice. For inmates, the collection of medication was a prized possession that was hoarded, traded for other capital, and used to develop medical records allowing them access to rights and resources in the community. Other objects were also obtained at the site of healthcare, and through their destruction, inmates and staff capitalised on a predictable infraction system that allowed them control over space and time in prison. Inmates' return to prison allowed them to re-enter a unique marketplace for benefits. Time in prison offered an escape from a chaotic life on the streets and a place of safety and security. The predictable routine of prison life allowed inmates the opportunity for emotional support and hope for the future. The prison was a place where inmates could detox from substance use and generate support by linking to community re-entry programmes and health and welfare systems by completing required paperwork and medical documentation.

Chapter 5 explores degradation from the perspective of staff, questioning their motives for actively degrading inmates. Staff came from the same community as offenders, built close relationships with them while "doing time" together, and depicted a similar dependence on the prison as a site for social change. Over time, prison staff found themselves drawn into a "tough" work culture where game playing was hard work. While officer training ensured that staff were physically able to maintain custody and control of inmates, it generally did not prepare them for the challenges of prison games. Union policies separated more experienced staff from inmates and contributed to some staff experiencing burnout. Staff expressed having little oversight in their daily work by senior supervisors and external evaluators. Staff, because of often shared biographical histories and relationships with inmates, degraded inmates to create a distance between themselves and the offender population. Staff attempted to create a level of distinction through conspicuous consumption and the policing of moral boundaries through punishment.

Chapter 6 continues to explore prison games from the perspective of staff and depicts how this group embodies a punishment regime over time. Staff were tasked with an impossible mission of offender rehabilitation and felt complicit when prison games undermined their efforts. This led the staff to feel that their work did not matter positively. Many staff expressed shame and emotional distress when delivering punishment to inmates. The staff did not feel emotionally supported, acknowledged, nor empowered by the prison administration. There was a dominant punishment culture in prison, which was at odds with care and rehabilitation. Colleagues saw staff who displayed care towards inmates as transgressing a punishment culture, and thus their actions were heavily policed.

Taken together, this study represents the lived experience of a group of HIV-positive inmates, as well as the people and institutions that framed their journey from prison to the community. This group of inmates, because of their healthcare needs, represents a particularly vulnerable population of offenders. On the one hand, an inmates HIV-positive status changed the field of prison games by opening more opportunities to gain capital in prison and during re-entry to the community. On the other hand, these individuals had a condition that required a high level of social and medical support, and without this support, they risked sickness and death. The prison was a site where health-vulnerable inmates could come and, however difficult, gain access to vital resources to improve their health and well-being.

Contextualising the Study Findings

The findings from this research should be considered alongside other prison literature. Criminologists have described how prison participants' narratives are shaped by the prison context (Crewe, 2007). Research participants may provide accounts that align themselves with expected institutional morals and practices. For example, inmates often depicted prison as a site to better their future by gaining access to resources, safety and security, healthcare, and other benefits. Inmates might have shared these narratives, in part, to explain transgressive behaviour and regular returns to prison. In this context, inmates sought to align themselves with an institution that, at least in theory, was meant to deliver rehabilitation services. Inmates often highlighted efforts to become reformed, placing any rehabilitative failure squarely on systems and institutions outside of their control. Similarly, staff depicted an unsupportive administration and pervasive culture of punishment in prison. These descriptions might have also been deployed to shift their responsibility for playing prison games on external factors outside their control. Interpretive challenges such as these were overcome by following analytical threads across different types of data, drawing from multiple participant accounts, and considering what was said alongside what was observed in the prison environment.

It is essential to consider that inmates played games in order to shift their identity from criminal to ill. This was why, in part, prison games were so heavily policed by prison staff at the site of healthcare. Other criminologists have made similar observations within the context of imprisonment (Davis & Shewan, 2000; Rhodes, 2004). Davis and

Shewan (2000) draw on drug use in prison to demonstrate how illness narratives were connected to an inmate's performance of "learned helplessness", whereby staff struggled to distinguish deliberate behavioural violations from serious illness. Rhodes (2004) made similar conclusions about the delivery of care to mentally ill offenders in a Washington State maximum-security prison. Her research draws on the tensions between rehabilitation and punishment, highlighting how prison staff regularly struggle to discern mental illness from "rational beings" in the context of imprisonment. Rhodes also recognised that inmates had exceptionally bounded agency under a punishment regime, describing solitary confinement as creating exceptional domination where inmates' only choice was to obey or resist an order, return a food tray, or throw faeces at staff (Rhodes, 2004). However, at least in the context of Melville, illness did not markedly divert inmates from criminal to ill. Although, having an illness did change the field of prison games for those living with HIV, as they had different access to healthcare providers and re-entry support. Nevertheless, inmates living with HIV were still required to play prison games as a quintessential feature of the prison environment. The stakes were exceptionally high for these individuals, as not receiving appropriate treatment could result in death.

Outside the prison setting, research on chronically ill hospital patients demonstrates that suffering legitimised a patient's entitlement to moral rights. A suffering sick person can make moral claims and have certain moral judgments conferred on him or her, such as deserving, dependent, or needing support (Charmaz, 1999). In Melville prison, the presentation of suffering from an illness did little to mitigate punishment and unlock better moral judgments from the staff. However, a certain level of suffering, or at least indisputable evidence of bodily damage, could legitimise claims under "deliberate indifference to a serious medical need" ("Estelle v. Gamble, 429 U.S. 97", 1976). Thus, suffering opened a pathway for inmates to access constitutionally mandated healthcare in the prison setting.

Prison games involved the production and use of violence in the context of imprisonment. Historically, the prevalence of "violence" has varied across prison institutions and has been reported differently for staff and inmates. For example, a study examining staff compensation claims in one U.S. jail found that half of all claims involved one or more violent clashes with inmates over a 10-year period (Safran & Tartaglinin, 1996). A systematic review by Dixon-Gordon, Harrison, and Roesch (2012) reported the prevalence of non-suicidal self-injury among inmates ranged from 7 to 48% of prisoners (Chapman, Specht, & Cellucci, 2005; Lader, Singleton, & Meltzer, 2003), with mentally disordered offenders experiencing even more violence in prison, ranging from 61 to 48% of prisoners (Gray et al., 2003; Loughran & Seewoonarain, 2005).

American prison literature has traditionally captured the prevalence and prediction of physical violence among the offender population (Byrne & Hummer, 2007; Kuanling, Sorensen, & Cunningham, 2008; Wolff, Blitz, Shi, Siegal, & Bachman, 2007; Wolff & Shi, 2011; Wolff, Vlitz, & Shi, 2007). This has included violence experienced by staff (Kartcoski, 1988; Safran & Tartaglinin, 1996), and descriptions of conceptual models to predict prison violence (Gadon, Johnstone, & Cooke, 2006; McCorkle, 1992; Sung, 2010; Wolff, Shi, & Blitz, 2007), as well as studies on how violence can be mitigated in prison settings (Cunningham & Sorensen, 2006; Medlicott, 2009). However, this literature has not traditionally explored the social constructs and structuring mechanisms that might produce prison violence. Instead, existing literature has focused on depicting physical assaults (Patrick, 1998; Wooldredge & Steiner, 2013), assaults between staff and inmates (Lahm, 2009; Patrick, 1998; Wolff et al., 2007), sexual assaults (Gaes & Goldberg, 2004; Jenness, Maxson, Matsuda, & Sumner, 2007), infliction of self-injury (Dixon-Gordon et al., 2012) and homicides and suicide among the offender population (Mumola, 2005).

European prison scholars addressing prison violence have given greater attention to the agency underpinning prison violence, particularly from inmates' perspective. Criminologists have interpreted prison violence as "necessary" for inmates and staff to redefine and renegotiate relationships in the prison setting (Edgar, O'Donnell, & Martin, 2003, p. 8). Others have described how violence is connected to the adaption and resistance of prison governance (Crewe, 2006, 2007). Crewe's research portrays how violence can exist as extreme acts and almost imperceptible social embodiments of resistance or what he describes as "displays of compliance that disguise oppositional objectives and hidden resistance" (Crewe,

2007, p. 271). These findings depict how power might be connected to a range of overt and subtle acts of resistance, and how these acts might be situationally produced through policies and prison management practices. Crewe (2007) has expanded what should be included when considering prison violence by accounting for both overt and organised resistance (Carrabine, 2004; Scraton, Sim, & Skidmore, 1991; Useem & Kimball, 1989), alongside other forms of violence such as hunger strikes, attempts of escape, and strategic use of legal actions and other political actions designed to undermine state power (Buntman, 2003; McEvoy, 2000).

Further, European prison scholars have described research findings supporting inmates' violent use of their bodies as a way of generating agency. This research details how inmates' use bodily fluids and self-harming behaviour to create political and social change (Feldman, 1991; Loughran, 1989; Yuill, 2007). This includes a description of "Dirty Protests" in Northern Ireland prisons as a site where inmates repurposed their bodies into political weapons by refusing to wash, smearing bodily excrement on cell walls, and carrying out hunger strikes (Yuill, 2007).

Representing the Study Findings

> Interpretive theory calls for the imaginative understanding of the studied phenomenon. This type of theory assumes emergent, multiple realities; indeterminacy; facts and values as linked; truth as provisional; and social life as processual. (Charmaz, 2006, pp. 126–127)

Constructivist grounded theory underpins this research, and so attention must be given to how this methodology frames the research findings. This methodology offered an inductive way of interpreting data to generate a theory about the prison environment. The analytical approach emphasises the importance of understanding a community of practice rather than seeking an explanation (Charmaz, 2006). Therefore, the theoretical understanding of degradation and prison games was something co-produced between the researcher and researched. This study also drew from Bourdieu's theory of practice when interpreting data. Thus, this study's analysis gives attention to how participant's biographies, engagement with one another, and structuring mechanisms created and informed a social practice of prison violence. The patterns and concepts presented in this book might apply to other members of the prison population and other prison settings in different ways. However, at least for those living with HIV in Melville and the staff who oversaw them, the experience of degradation and prison games was a part of everyday life.

In order to represent the agentic qualities of violence in the context of imprisonment, it was essential to step back and explore the consequences of violent acts both at the time they occurred in prison and after the offender returned to the community. It was also crucial to breakdown categorical lines of victim and perpetrator, as well as the oppressor and the oppressed, to consider how violence was co-produced and used across people in different positions of power. Violence was a delicate thing in prison, on the one hand agency producing, and on the other hand, highly destructive and interpreted differently by members of the prison community.

Writing about violence can create a degree of violence. Labelling and identifying what is and is not violent expands this concept in new ways, shifts responsibility on people and institutions, and can be subjugating for those who experience it (Bourgois, 2001). Das, Kleinman, Ramphele, and Reynolds (2000) suggest that the act of writing on violence is a task that haunts many ethnographers who study it (Das et al., 2000). However, this in no way means we should turn away from the study of violence, but instead offer thoughtful accounts of how individuals and collective groups experience violence from different perspectives and in different contexts (Das et al., 2000). Further, understanding violence as potentially productive and contiguous with everyday social relations, as has been shown in this study, does not necessarily mean it is morally virtuous. Rather it points to a more nuanced way of theorising the "constructive and preservation motivations and meanings violence can have in different contexts" (Jauregui, 2013, p. 12).

Further, it is important to be clear that the research findings from this study were derived through a specific qualitative methodology, and claims made in this book only represent one state prison system at a point in time. Thus, the findings should be considered alongside other research considering the American prison experience and comparisons drawn to other national contexts.

Improving American Prisons

This book leaves readers with several unanswered questions about what can be done to change prison games and reimprisonment patterns among offenders living with HIV. How can healthcare, justice, and welfare interventions build on bounded agency in prison without creating more violence? Can the production of prison games be undone? How can such a systemic, structural, recursive process such as prison games be diverted, or is it inevitable so long as the prison exists? How can interventions seek to absorb the harms of degradation and prison games to protect inmates and staff from becoming complicit in their enactment? In fact, what are the implications of access to healthcare for those in need of treatment and care for HIV?

While these questions require further research on the experience of HIV-positive offenders at all stages of their involvement in the criminal justice system, it is possible to look to other countries for models that might alleviate some of the violent conditions described in this book.

Reform for HIV-Positive Offenders

HIV-positive offenders were required to engage in prison games to access healthcare and capital in prison and position themselves for better welfare and health support upon return to the community. Once discharged from the prison, these individuals often faced disrupted healthcare and welfare (e.g., delayed Medicaid), which was further complicated by structural drivers. Findings from this study suggest that even despite prison games, reimprisonment might offer an escape from a chaotic life in the community, inspired by feelings of isolation and anonymity; the stress of overexertion from social forces and responsibilities; and familiarity with the prison context. Prison offered a place of safety and security from other types of violence brought on by troubled social networks and inadequate community healthcare. Through its routinised structure, the prison offered inmates time to concentrate on their health and well-being and to avoid certain types of stigma more pronounced in the community. Incarceration provided an intervention for persons struggling with addiction, who had trouble securing long-term treatment through community care. It offered renewed opportunities to access support structures intended to transition individuals to become independent community members.

Nevertheless, inmates' return to prison as a solution to health and social problems has deleterious social and fiscal consequences that transcend social stratum. For the readmitted offender, this included a further criminal record, fractured community ties, lost resources, disrupted treatment, and the loss of liberties. It demanded their engagement in a prison marketplace that required escalating acts of violence and the playing of prison games to gain access to healthcare and welfare benefits. However, there are also costs to the public, which might include the maintenance of a vast criminal justice system, where the prison structure incurs costs related to operations (e.g., personnel salaries), infrastructure, transportation, food, education, as well as rehabilitative programming and healthcare for a growing population with significant health needs. On average, U.S. states spend over $33,000 per inmate, per year, nationwide (Mai & Subramanian, 2017). There are further costs associated with policing, victims, juridical proceedings, probation and parole, families and social networks disrupted or left behind. Reports attempting to quantify the total cost of U.S. incarceration have provided figures as high as $182 Billion per year (Wagner & Rabuy, 2017).

Where offenders have a chronic illness such as HIV, the underlying problem will remain unaddressed as the reimprisonment cycle is set to repeat itself until individuals receive comprehensive public support and care or die. Previous studies described significant disruptions in HIV care for inmates returning from prison to community settings (Baillargeon, 2009). Critical to achieving HIV viral suppression is linking individuals into care and retaining them in treatment. Research has shown that for those who do successfully link to care upon release, they are 24 to 29% less likely to continue treatment when compared to those who are not involved in the criminal justice system (Costa, 2018). Further, HIV incidence is highest in detainees released and re-incarcerated when compared with continuously incarcerated prisoners (Dolan, 2016). Considering people in prison are five times more likely to be living with HIV than the general population, these circumstances create a public health risk to the general prisoner population and as the disadvantaged communities from which prisons disproportionately draw (Clear, 2007).

This evidence raises the question of criminal justice reform in America and how we might consider non-prison-based healthcare and welfare programming in and around a system of "mass imprisonment". This study's findings highlight the need for a single-payer healthcare system to better support those living with HIV and leaving prison. However, the U.S. continues to find itself in the situation where imprisonment remains the only setting where citizens have a constitutional right to medical care, thus creating a prison healthcare system delivered separately from the general population. While universal healthcare is not presently a reality in the U.S., the ACA has taken substantial steps towards achieving greater equal access to healthcare for Americans, which has led numerous states to enrol inmates into community healthcare prior to their release (Bandara, 2015). However, further research is needed to understand how prison and non-prison healthcare systems connect and deliver healthcare services. Similarly, there is a need to understand the factors that affect health-vulnerable offenders' decisions to access healthcare in the community, as well as perceptions of health and health care in the re-entry process. This will become increasingly important as access to medical care improves in the U.S. Yet, we might start by looking at how single-payer healthcare systems have evolved in Australia (Medicaid) and Britain (NHS) for guidance on how to address the practicalities of transitional prison to community care against the backdrop of large carceral populations.

The data from this study also highlights a need to consider the cultural beliefs that underpin different social and welfare drivers for the reimprisonment of HIV-positive offenders. Prison systems in Nordic states—Finland, Norway, and Sweden—provide examples of nations with low imprisonment rates for comparison. Nordic cultures support welfare through communal values for solidarity, social structures, and egalitarianism, which, in part, has enabled the avoidance of mass imprisonment altogether (Pratt, 2008a, b). Pratt argues the cultural basis of many of these factors means that they are not always transferable to other nations. However, the Nordic model warrants attention for suggesting how, specifically in cultures with proportionally larger prison populations, we might consider narratives of degradation and prison games and reimprisonment to shift underlying orthodoxies that support mass imprisonment. Here, the research findings move the discussion away from the common response of "punishment vs. rehabilitation" when addressing transgressive behaviour, and instead suggest that we must address a situation where people feel compelled to use the prison system to gain access to specific rights and resources that would be more appropriately and inexpensively delivered in public settings.

Reform for Prison Staff

Staff are critical to the operation of safe, secure, and humane prisons, yet are often missing or reductively portrayed in the literature (Bennett, Crewe, & Wahidin, 2008; Liebling & Price, 2001). Liebling (2000) describes prison staff as the "invisible ghosts of penality" (Liebling, 2000, p. 337). Similarly, Crewe et al. (2008) draws attention to how traditional sociological accounts "depict guards as shadowy figures, peripheral to the main action, and who are just there as an inertial and conservative influence" (Sparks et al. 1996, as cited in Crewe, 2008, p.3). Crewe et al. describe that historically, when prison officers have been illustrated in prison literature, they are deleteriously depicted as "ghoulish figures, facelessly patrolling the landings, obstructing researchers or enforcing their power in monolithically authoritarian ways" (Crewe, Bennett, & Wahidin, 2008, p. 2). Thus, it is not surprising that many prison staff often see themselves as neglected and unappreciated (Crawley, 2004; Thomas, 1972).

However, prison scholars have more recently started to include staff in research. Roy, Novak, and Miksaj-Todorovic (2010) outlines this body of literature, which includes accounts of general prison staff, custodial staff, and who provide other types of services such as education, work training, healthcare, and leisure time activities (Roy et al., 2010). This literature describes how the prison environment affects staff's the emotional well-being, which in turn brings about increased stress among them, affects job satisfaction, and results in high levels of burnout. (Arnold, 2005; Garland, 2002; Garland, Lambert, Hogan, Kim, & Kelley, 2014; Miksaj-Todorovic & Novak, 2008; Slade & Lopresti, 2013; Stack & Tsoudis, 1997).

This study does not wish to contribute to a negative portrayal of prison staff nor leave them unaccounted for in the ethnographic account. Instead, the research findings point to how staff might struggle to cope in a context where there is little social separation from themselves and the offender population. The research findings suggest that U.S. prison staff embrace a hardened punishment regime, characterised by extreme sanctions such as solitary confinement. The study also finds that carrying out punishment is difficult for staff and supersedes any attempt at delivering proactive care and rehabilitation. Therefore, we must take a targeted approach to equip staff to deliver rehabilitation in prisons better and improve their job satisfaction, health, and well-being.

European prisons have seen a "rehabilitation resurgence" in recent decades (Robinson & Crow, 2009; Sumramanian & Shames, 2013) and offer comparison sites. The U.K. and the Netherlands have reformed the role of staff when developing models offender rehabilitation. These two nations address offenders with mental health challenges and offer promising pathways to improve the experience of staff and the relational environment in prison.

The U.K. has taken an innovative approach to offender rehabilitation by creating Psychologically Informed Planned Environments (PIPE), a part of the Offender Personality Disorder Pathway (Benefield, Turner, Bolger, & Bainbridge, 2017; Bennett, 2014). PIPEs are structured and planned environments where the staff is trained to deliver a psychologically informed offender management approach. As such, staff are required to develop a supportive relationship with offenders and model pro-social behaviour (Turley, Payne, & Webster, 2013). PIPEs are not treatment interventions, but instead offer a space with augmented support for inmates to transition through significant stages of imprisonment (National Offender Management Service & Department of

Health, 2012). In practice, prison staff facilitate structured groups with inmates and creative sessions, which are carried out alongside training, supervision, and reflection (Turley et al., 2013). The PIPE aims to provide an environment that facilitates healthy relationships, encourages inmates to engage in positive social behaviour, and encourages all prison members to take responsibility for themselves, others, and the shared prison environment (Turley et al., 2013). Early empirical research on PIPEs shows that this model creates a positive relational setting and improves relationships between staff and inmates (Castledine, 2015).

Another European model that has changed the role of staff to facilitate rehabilitation is the Dutch approach to imprisonment. This model diverts the most problematic offenders with mental health issues into secure forensic health hospitals and outpatient clinics (De Boer, Whyte, & Maden, 2008). This pathway includes *Terugdringen Recidive* correctional facilities (TR; "Reducing Recidivism"), which falls under *Terbeschikkingstelling* (TBS; "At The Disposal of The Government") (De Boer et al., 2008). In TR settings, staff are trained to deliver mental health support and work with offenders to transition them to life in the community. Crucially, this system identifies and channels ill offenders into alternative Court systems that, in turn, place offenders in appropriate healthcare settings. This process enables mentally challenged offenders to access appropriate treatment and rehabilitation services (Badley, 2009; McRae, 2015). This approach to offender rehabilitation has, in part, led to a sustained reduction in new criminal convictions and recidivism (Ministry of Security and Justice, 2011).

Presently, there is a need for new research into how staff might transition from a supervisor or guard to a multi-skilled manager, and how this change in role and responsibility might impact their health, well-being, and job satisfaction. However, there is increasing evidence that this change can be positive for both staff and inmates. Not addressing the experience of prison staff will inevitably lead to failed rehabilitation and the continuation of a prison punishment paradigm.

Inmates face substantial barriers to their successful transition to public life, as imprisonment is a limited degrading marketplace for health and welfare resources. It is my impression that both staff and inmates have the potential to contribute to the "common good". However, significant structural and social obstacles must be resolved to achieve this, and a better rehabilitation model adopted. To this end, further research into HIV-positive person's experiences in other prison settings is required. This should be done with consideration for how different institutions and values might reciprocally shape the act of imprisonment and draw comparisons across a diversity of carceral settings. From this, new interventions and policies must be developed.

References

Arnold, H. (2005). The effects of prison work. In A. Liebling & S. Maruna (Eds.), *The effects of imprisonment* (pp. 391–420). Cullomption, UK: Willan

Badley, K. (2009). *Lord bradley's review of people with mental health problems or learning disabilities in the criminal justice system* (The Bradley Report). Retrieved from: https://webarchive.nationalarchives.gov.uk/20130105193845/http://www.dh.gov.uk/prod_consum_dh/groups/dh_digitalassets/documents/digitalasset/dh_098698.pdf.

Baillargeon, J., Giordano, T. P., Rich, J. D., Wu, Z. H., Wells, K., Pollock, B. H., & Paar, D. P. (2009). Accessing antiretroviral therapy following release from prison. *Journal of the American Medical Association, 301*(8), 848–857.

Bandara, S. N., Huskamp, H. A., Riedel, L. E., McGinty, E. E., Webster, D., Toone, R. E., & Barry, C. L. (2015). Leveraging the affordable care act to enroll justice-involved populations in medicaid: State and local efforts. *Health Affairs, 34*(12), 2044–2051.

Benefield, N., Turner, K., Bolger, L., & Bainbridge, C. (2017). *Psychogically informed planned envionments—A new optimism for criminal justice provision?* (Unpublished Manuscript).

Bennett, A. L. (2014). Service users' initial hopes, expectations and experiences of a high security psychologically informed planned environment (PIPE). *Journal of Forensic Pratice, 16*(3), 216–227.

Bennett, J., Crewe, B., & Wahidin, A. (2008). *Understanding prison staff*. Cullompton, UK: Willan.

Bourgois, P. (2001). The power of violence in war and peace. *Ethnography, 2*(1), 5–34.

Buntman, F. L. (2003). *Robben island and prisoner resistance to apartheid.* Cambridge, UK: Cambridge University Press.

Byrne, J. M., & Hummer, D. (2007). Myths and realities of violence: A review of the evidence. *Victims & Offenders, 2*(1), 77–90.
Carrabine, E. (2004). *Power, discourse and resistance: A genealogy of the strangeways prison riot.* Dartmouth: Ashgate.
Castledine, S. (2015). Psychologically informed and planned environments: A community perspective. *Probation Journal, 62*(3), 273–280.
Chapman, A., Specht, M. W., & Cellucci, T. (2005). Borderline personality disorder and deliberate self-harm: Does experiential avoidance play a role? *Suicide and Life-Threatening Behavior,* (35), 388–399.
Charmaz, K. (1999). Stories of suffering: Subjective tales of research narratives. *Qualitative Health Research, 9*(3), 362–382.
Charmaz, K. (2006). *Constructing grounded theory: A practical guide through qualitative analysis.* London, UK: Sage Publications.
Clear, T. R. (2007). *Imprisoning communities: How mass incarceration makes disadvantaged neighborhoods worse.* Oxford and New York: Oxford University Press.
Costa, M., Montague, B. T., Solomon, L., Sammartino, C., Gutman, R., Zibman, C., Rosen, D., & Rich, J. D. (2018). Assessing the effect of recent incarceration in prison on HIV care retention and viral suppression in two states. *Journal of Urban Health, 95*(4), 499–507.
Crawley, E. (2004). *Doing prison work: The public and private lives of prison officers.* Cullompton, UK: Willan
Crewe, B. (2006). *The prison society: Power, adaptation, and social life in an English prison.* Oxford, UK: Oxford University Press.
Crewe, B. (2007). Power, adaptation and resistance in a late-modern men's prison. *British Journal of Crimonology, 47*, 256–275.
Crewe, B., Bennett, J., & Wahidin, A. (2008). Introduction. In J. Bennett, B. Crewe, & A. Wahidin (Eds.), *Understanding prison staff* (pp. 1–11). Cullompton, UK and Portland, OR: Willan.
Cunningham, M. D., & Sorensen, J. R. (2006). Actuarial models for assessing prison violence risk: Revisions and extensions of the risk assessment scale for prison (RASP). *Assessment, 13*(253).
Das, V., Kleinman, A., Ramphele, M., & Reynolds, P. (2000). *Violence and subjectivity.* Berkeley, CA: University of California Press.
Davis, J. B., & Shewan, D. (2000). The macro and micro logic of drug and prisons. In J. B. Davis & D. Shewan (Eds.), *An international perspective.* Amsterdam, NL: Harwood Academic Publishers.
De Boer, J., Whyte, S., & Maden, T. (2008). Compulsory treatment of dangerous offenders with severe personility disorders: A comparison of the

English DSPD and Dutch TBS systems. *The Journal of Forensic Psychiatry & Psychology, 19*(2), 148–163.

Dixon-Gordon, K., Harrison, N., & Roesch, R. (2012). Non-suicidal self-injury within offender populations: A systematic review. *International Journal of Forensic Mental Health, 11*, 30–50.

Dolan, K., Wirtz, A. L., Moazen, B., Ndeffo-Mbah, M., Galvani, A., Kinner, … Altice, F. L. (2016). Global burden of HIV, viral hepatitis, and tuberculosis in prisoners and detainees. *Lancet, 388*, 1089–1102.

Edgar, K., O'Donnell, I., & Martin, C. (2003). *Prison violence: The dynamics of conflict, fear and power*. New York, NY: Routledge.

Estelle v. Gamble, 429 U.S. 97, 97 426 (Supreme Court of the United States 1976).

Feldman, A. (1991). *Formations of violence: The narraitives of the body and political terror in Northern Ireland*. Chicago, IL: University of Chicago.

Gadon, L., Johnstone, L., & Cooke, D. (2006). Situational variables and institutional violence: A systematic review of the literature. *Clinical Psychology Review, 26*, 515–534.

Gaes, G. G., & Goldberg, A. (2004). *Prison rape: A critical review of the literature*. National Institute of Justice: Washington, DC. Retrieved from: https://www.ncjrs.gov/pdffiles1/nij/grants/213365.pdf.

Garland, B. (2002). Prison treatment staff burnout: Consequences, causes, and prevention *Corrections Today, 64*(7), 116–121.

Garland, B., Lambert, E. G., Hogan, N. L., Kim, B., & Kelley, T. (2014). The relationship of affective and continuance organisational commitment with correctional staff occupational burnout—A partial replication and expansion study. *Criminal Justice & Behavior, 41*(10), 1161–1177.

Gray, N. S., Hill, C., McGleish, A., Timmons, D., MacCulloch, M. J., & Snowden, R. J. (2003). Prediction of violence and self-harm in mentally disordered offenders: A prospective study of the efficacy of HCR-20, PCL-R, and psychiatric symptomatology. *Journal of Consulting and Clinical Psychology, 71*(3), 443–451.

Jauregui, B. (2013). Dirty anthropology: Epistemologies of violence and ethical entanglements in police ethnography. In W. Garriott (Ed.), *Policing and contemporary governance: The anthropology of police in pratice*. New York, NY: Palgrave Macmillan.

Jenness, V., Maxson, K. N., Matsuda, K. N., Sumner, J. M. (2007). *Violence in California correctional facilities: An emperical examination of sexual assault*. Center for Evidence-Based Corrections, University of California, Irvine:

Irvine, CA. Retrieved from: https://www.prearesourcecenter.org/sites/default/files/library/55-preapresentationpreareportucijennessetal.pdf.
Kartcoski, P. C. (1988). The implications of research explaining prison violence and disruption. *Federal Probation, 52*(1), 27–32.
Kuanling, A., Sorensen, J. R., & Cunningham, M. D. (2008). Juvenile inmates in an adult prison system: Rates of disciplinary misconduct and violence. *Criminal Justice and Behavior,* (35), 1186.
Lader, D., Singleton, N., & Meltzer, H. (2003). Psychiatric morbidity among young offenders in England and Wales. *International Review of Psychiatry,* (15), 144–147.
Lahm, K. F. (2009). Inmate assaults on prison staff A multilevel examination of an overlooked form of prison violence. *Criminology and Penology, 89*(2), 131–150.
Liebling, A., & Price, D. (2001). *The Prison Officer.* HMP Leyhill, UK: Prison Servicce Journal.
Loughran, C. (1989). Armagh and feminist strategy: Campaigns around republican women prisoners in armagh jail. *Feminist Review,* (23), 59–79.
Loughran, M., & Seewoonarain, K. (2005). Characteristics of need and risk among women prisoners referred to inreach mental health services. *The British Journal of Forensic Practice, 7*, 12–21.
Mai, C., & Subramanian, R. (2017). *Price of prisons 2015: Examining state spending trends, 2010–2015.* Vear Institute of Justice: New York, NY. Retrieved from: https://www.vera.org/publications/price-of-prisons-2015-state-spending-trends.
McCorkle, R. C. (1992). Personal precautions to violence in prison. *Criminal Justice and Behavior, 19*(2), 160–173.
McEvoy, K. (2000). *Paramilitary imprisonment in Northern Ireland*. Oxford: Clarendon Press.
McRae, L. (2015). The offender personality disorder pathway: Risking rehabilitation? *Medical Law Review, 23*(3), 321–347.
Medlicott, D. (2009). Preventing torture and casual cruelty in prisons through independent monitoring. In P. Scranton & J. McCulloch (Eds.), *The violence of incarceration.* New York, NY: Routledge
Miksaj-Todorovic, L., & Novak, T. (2008). Research of emotional well-being and job burnout of prison staff. *kriminologija i socijalna intergracija, 16*(1), 1–126.
Ministry of Security and Justice. (2011). *Recidivism report 2002–2008.* The Hague. Retrieved from: https://www.wodc.nl/binaries/factsheet-2011-5a-def-4apr2012-mk_tcm28-71815.pdf.

Mumola, C. (2005). *Suicide and homicide in state prisons and local jails.* U.S. Bureau of Justice Statistics: Washington, DC. Retrieved from: https://www.bjs.gov/content/pub/pdf/shsplj.pdf.

National Offender Management Service & Department of Health. (2012). *A guide to psychologically informed planned environments.* London: National Offender Management Service and Department of Health.

Patrick, S. (1998). Differences in inmate and inmate-staff altercations: Examples from a medium security prison. *The Social Science Journal, 35*(2), 253–263.

Pratt, J. (2008a). Scandinavian exceptionalism in an era of penal excess; Part I: The nature and roots of scandinavian exceptionalism. *The British Journal of Criminology, 48*, 119–137.

Pratt, J. (2008b). Scandinavian exceptionalism in an era of penal excess; Part II: Does scandinavian exceptionalism have a future? *British Journal of Criminology, 48*, 275–292.

Rhodes, L. A. (2004). *Total confinement: Madness and reason in the maximum security prison.* Berkeley, CA: University of California Press.

Robinson, G., & Crow, I. D. (2009). *Offender rehabilitation theory, research and practice*. London, UK: Sage.

Roy, S., Novak, T., & Miksaj-Todorovic. (2010). Job burnout among prison staff in the United States and Croatia: A preliminary comparative study. *International Journal of Criminal Justice Sciences, 5*(1), 189–202.

Safran, D. A., & Tartaglinin, A. J. (1996). Workplace violence in an urban jail setting. In G. R. VandenBos & E. Q. Bulatao (Eds.), *Violence on the job: Identifying risks and developing solutions.* Washington, DC: American Psycological Association.

Scraton, P., Sim, J., & Skidmore, P. (1991). *Prisons under protest*. Milton Keynes: Open University Press.

Slade, K., & Lopresti, S. (2013). *Promoting resilience in prison staff*. Nottingham, UK. Retrieved from: http://irep.ntu.ac.uk/id/eprint/2343/1/216927_PubSub642Slade.pdf.

Stack, S., & Tsoudis, O. (1997). Suicide risk among correctional officers: A logistical regression analysis. *Archives of Sucide Research, 3*(3), 183–186.

Sumramanian, R., & Shames, A. (2013). *Sentencing and prison practices in Germany and the Netherlands: Implications for the United States.* Vera Institute of Justice: New York, NY. Retrieved from: https://www.vera.org/publications/sentencing-and-prison-practices-in-germany-and-the-netherlands-implications-for-the-united-states.

Sung, H.-E. (2010). Prevalence and risk factors of violence-related and accident-related injuries among state prisoners. *Journal of Correctional Health Care, 16*(3), 178–187.

Thomas, J. E. (1972). *The English prison officer since 1850: A study in conflict.* London, UK: Routledge & Kegan Paul Books.

Turley, C., Payne, C., & Webster, S. (2013). *Enabling features of psychologically informed planned environments.* London: Ministry of Justice.

Useem, B., & Kimball, P. (1989). *States of Siege: US prison riots, 1971–1986*. Oxford, UK: Oxford University Press.

Wagner, P., & Rabuy, B. (2017). *Following the money of mass incarceration.* Prison Policy Initative: Northampton, MA. Retrieved from: https://www.prisonpolicy.org/reports/money.html.

Wolff, N., Blitz, C. L., Shi, J., Siegal, J., & Bachman, R. (2007). Physical violence inside prisons: Rates of victimization. *Criminal Justice and Behavior, 34*(5), 588–599.

Wolff, N., & Shi, J. (2011). Patterns of victimization and feelings of safty inside prison: The experience of male and female inmates. *Crime & Delinquency, 57*, 29.

Wolff, N., Shi, J., & Blitz, C. L. (2007). Racial and ethnic disparities in types of sources of victimization inside prison. *The Prison Journal, 2*(1), 77–90.

Wolff, N., Vlitz, C. L., & Shi, J. (2007). Rates of sexual victimization in prison for inmates with and without mental disorders. *Psychiatric Services, 58*(8), 1087.

Wooldredge, J., & Steiner, B. (2013). Violent victimization among sate prison inmates. *Violence and Victims, 28*(3), 531–551.

Yuill, C. (2007). The body as weapon: Bobby sands and the republican hunger strikes. *Sociological Research Online, 12*(2). Retrieved from http://www.socresonline.org.uk/12/2/yuill.html.

Appendix A: Study Design

The research study drew from constructivist grounded theory (Charmaz, 2003, 2006), and thus maintained a broad focus on "what was going on" in prison and peri-carceral space. This involved carrying out concurrent fieldwork and analysis in order to work towards generating a theory of practice. Analytic codes and categories emerged from data, not preconceived hypotheses, which guided further data collection and analytical interpretations. This involved making ongoing comparisons across different types of data (interview transcripts, fieldnotes, and documents) and relevant literature throughout the duration of the study (Charmaz, 2006, pp. 5–6). Emerging data was regularly "fractured" in order to establish themes. Themes were followed up with new questions, refined topic guides, and included different spaces and participants (Green & Thorogood, 2009, p. 203). The research was initially guided by a set of research questions, including: What is the experience of HIV-positive inmates as they move from prison to the community?; How do medical and security staff negotiate positions with inmates in the correctional setting?; How do systems of punishment, rehabilitation, and health and welfare shape participants lives?

L. Kuester, *Violence in Pursuit of Health*, Palgrave Studies in Prisons and Penology, https://doi.org/10.1007/978-3-030-61350-1

Data collection methods comprised semi-structured interviews and participant observations. This took place across six overlapping research segments from 2011 to 2013 (Fig. A.1: Research segments). The research segments were intended to capture a diversity of participants' lived experiences as they journeyed through incarceration. However, the unpredictable nature of incarceration meant that a segmented study design was only used as a loose guide, as several participants unexpectedly incarcerated during the duration of this study.

Participant Eligibility

All interview participants were 18 years of age or older, demonstrated proficient English language, and consented to participate. Inmate and ex-inmate participant's spent time in prison and tested positive for HIV. Inmates and ex-inmates had the option of inviting a family member, partner, or caregiver (18 years of age or older) to participate in a community follow-up interview, provided consent was obtained. Prison and community professionals were required to be employed by the prison system or have carried out work associated with the criminal justice system, either in healthcare or social support.

Fieldwork Segments

Ethical permissions were obtained, and background checks completed prior to entering the research field. I was granted "Green level" security clearance, which allowed unescorted entry to most state jail and prison facilities.

Segment 1: Building Relationships. On 27 October 2011, rapport was established with research participants. Several participant observation activities commenced in prison (e.g., exercise class with offenders and observing HIV clinic) and community settings (e.g., observing case management support). Activities started in this phase continued throughout the study.

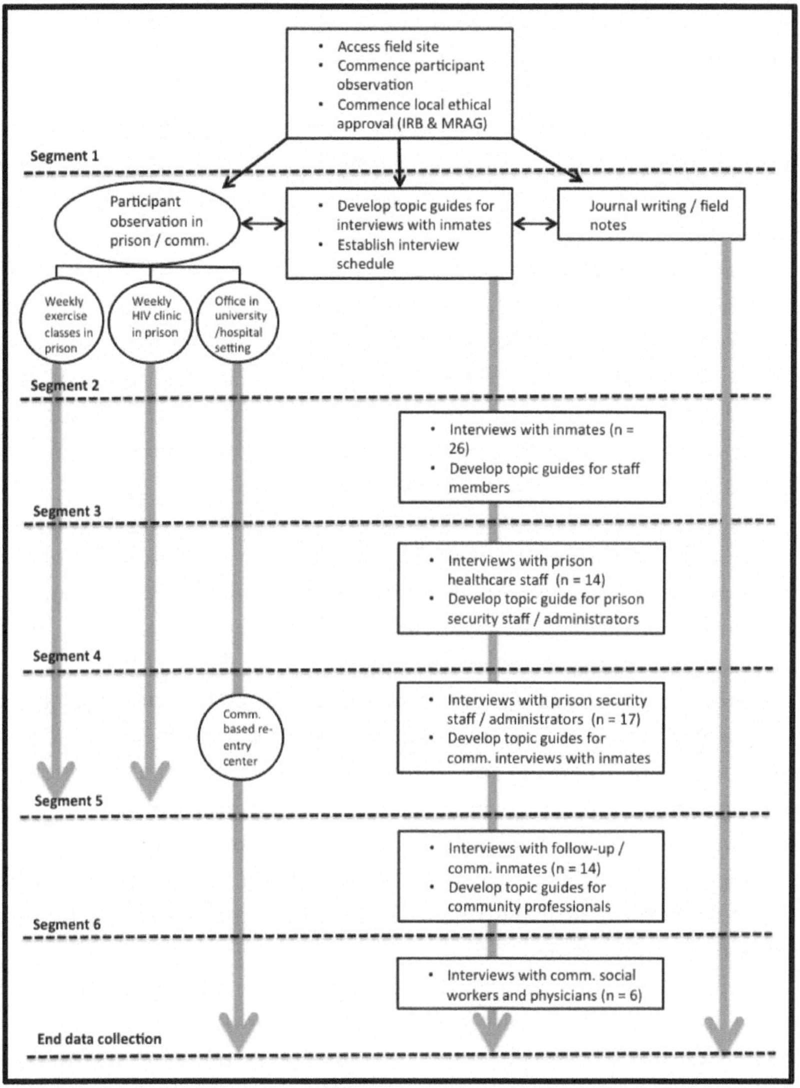

Figure A.1 Segments of research

Segment 2: Inmate Interviews. On 16 February 2012, interviews with short and long-term inmates living with HIV (n = 26) commenced in prison. Short-term inmates were inmates' expecting to leave the prison within 1 year from the interview date, whereas long-term inmates were considered inmates' serving 1 year or longer at the time of the interview. A set of four topic guides were developed and refined during this segment of research.

Segment 3: Healthcare Staff Interviews. On 30 April 2012, interviews with prison healthcare staff (n = 14) commenced in prison. A prison education programme was established, and observational work on a State Taskforce for HIV Prevention was undertaken at this time. A joint prison-academic course was also launched. Interview topic guides for security professionals were refined, and a study amendment to include inmate's partners, family, and caregivers was made.

Segment 4: Officer Interviews. On 24 May 2012, interviews with prison officers and administrators (n = 17) commenced in prison. Increasing time was spent observing community-based inmate re-entry support programmes for HIV-positive offenders (AIDS Resource Centre). Topic guides for community-based follow-up interviews were refined.

Segment 5: Ex-inmate Interviews. On 24 July 2012, follow-up interviews with short-term inmates leaving prison (n = 14) commenced at ARC and in other community settings. This also included interviewing family, partners, and caregivers of justice-involved individuals living with HIV. Ex-inmates who had been living in the community for one year or longer were also recruited to participate in the study through ARC. Twenty-nine parole hearings were observed. Topic guides for community professionals were refined.

Segment 6: Community Health Interviews. On 10 September 2012, interviews with community-based outreach workers, social workers, project managers, and HIV medical consultants (n = 6) commenced in a range of community settings.

Interviews

Informed consent was obtained before each interview. Interviews were audio recorded and transcribed. Topic guides were used to keep interviews on track, but participants were encouraged to take the lead during conversations. Individual topic guides were developed for inmates, prison staff, follow-up interviews, ex-inmates in the community, and community-based staff. Developing guides was a recursive process throughout the duration of the study. Often, amendments to guides were made by scribbling notes in the margins during interviews, crossing out questions, adding new questions, and flagging questions to return to later. Fieldnote journals were kept throughout the study, and these notes were used to tailor questions to individual participants. As analytical themes emerged through on-going data analysis, topic guides were refined to follow analytical threads.

The questions within the guides were open-ended and intended to encourage unanticipated statements and stories to emerge from research the participant's accounts (Charmaz, 2006, p. 26). Guides were organised around domains intended to elicit narratives about participant's lives in prison and the community. For example, the topic guide for inmates included questions about social relationships, interaction with staff, experience living with HIV, life events, past social relationships, and expectations for the future.

Participants were encouraged to go off-topic, interrupt a line of questioning, and discuss topics they felt were more important or relevant. Often, I asked participants to clarify or elaborate responses by providing examples. Throughout the study, I presented emerging themes to participants and asked them to explain or challenge my initial interpretations.

Topic guides were not uniformly used across all participants. For example, some senior staff had limited time to complete interviews, and therefore fewer questions were explored with these participants. Every effort was made to accommodate participant's schedules, which meant interviews were sometimes conducted across multiple sittings. Interviews with inmates were carried out in a range of confidential spaces, utilising empty clinical rooms, chapels, and visitation centres within prison facilities. Staff meetings and community-based interviews took place in a venue of the participants choosing. While financial incentives were prohibited in the prison setting, a $10.00 cash incentive was provided to participants taking part in a community-based follow-up interview.

Participant Observation

To be specific about the type of account represented in this research, it is important to be clear about my position as "observer-as-participant" (Atkinson & Hammersley, 1994, p. 249). Hong and Duff (2002) offer a guide to establishing ethnographic immersion, which has been mapped across four distinct phases: "initiation", the preliminary observation of the research setting; "understanding", the first one-to-one conversations with participants; "acceptance", the spontaneous expression of comments and opinions by participants, and; "trust", which happens when participants become at ease with the researcher (Hong & Duff, 2002).

During "initiation", which occurred before formal interviews, I developed a rapport with inmates through informal conversations on the MOD (wing) and individual cells. I also watched TV, observed HIV clinic, and regularly exercised with inmates. I informally talked with staff in healthcare settings and security substations. Later, in the community, this also included observing client consultations at the AIDS Resource Centre and Melville Hospital, as well as shadowing social workers during client home visits, appointments at welfare offices, and observations at other offender rehabilitation services.

Early in the study, I noticed that the staff appeared to be suspicious of my presence in the institution. They compared my role to visitors, medical consultants, lawyers, and generally "outsiders" who regularly moved through the prison but didn't seek to integrate into the institution's day-to-day routine. Fieldnotes documented how staff initially shouted to their colleagues to "keep quiet while this guy is around", or "watch out, he's keeping notes on us".

Therefore, it was important to be seen spending time in prison. Time enabled me to develop "understanding". "Doing time" was critical to becoming an insider. Whether as a staff member or resident, participating in monotonous, routine, and lonely periods of time demonstrated commitment and understanding of a shared experience of incarceration. At the beginning of the research, I regularly spent 5 days per week, and 7 to 12 hours a day moving between facilities and engaging with different members of the prison community.

To "do time", I scheduled interviews to coincide with what was referred to as "deadtime". Deadtime occurred when movement in a facility was restricted, ranging from a few hours to an entire day. Movement restrictions were put in place when officers needed to conduct a count,[1] a facility went into lockdown,[2] or during inmate chow and recreation. While scheduling interviews during this time often created delays in leaving the prison and moving freely, it also meant that staff and inmates would have more time to talk while most activities were suspended. This enabled me to advance towards "acceptance", a phase characterised by established trust with participants. Participants began to share their biographical stories, expressing opinions, sharing institutional secrets, and seeing me as part of the fabric of the prison community.

I connected with staff by discussing football, goat farming, civil war history, sports cars, etc. I would note their interests in fieldnotes and read about the topics that interested them (Janes, 1969, p. 56). Six months into fieldwork, I gained increasing "acceptance" by staff. Officers invited me to attend drinks after work. Healthcare staff would ask that I keep them company while doing routine tasks, such as reviewing medical slips. Furthermore, the Brass (senior officers) welcomed my presence, and I was invited to spend more time talking with these participants in security substations and administrative offices. For example, one senior officer arranged to have an extra food tray delivered to the wing so we could eat together. Acceptance from staff enabled greater freedom to move around the institution, particularly within more high-security facilities.

---

[1]Human inventory of the prison. Counts occurred 6 times per day at 5:00 am, 10:30 am, 3:15 pm, 9:00 pm, and 2:00 am.

[2]Lockdown is the restriction of inmate movement. This was result of a code being called (e.g., code blue was used for a security breach, and code white was used for a medical emergency) or staffing shortages. Throughout the study, there were over 157 lockdowns across the prison institution.

This allowed for more time with inmates, and engaging in activities such as playing card games, exercise, and art projects. This level of acceptance allowed for my account of prison life to be more line with a "participant as an observer".

My role in the community of practice might be considered "moderate participation" (Spradley, 1980, p. 60), as "complete participation", such as being imprisoned or working as an officer was not possible, nor do I believe it would have been an ethically appropriate role as a researcher. Tables A.1, A.2, A.3, A.4, and A.5 provide a full listing of participant observation activities carried out during research.

Table A.1 Inmate participant observation

Population/participants	Activity	Location	Duration/frequency
Female inmates	I ran an exercise class fir inmate in the prison. Participants received "meritorious goodtime" for participating	Women's facilities (prison yard and visiting hall)	Twice weekly (segment 1–5)
HIV-positive inmates, nurses, medical consultants	I observed 250 clinical consultations between inmates and their HIV specialist	All prison facilities (medical dispensary)	Half-day clinics that were offered twice weekly (segment 1–5)
Female inmates, state officials, prison administrators, wardens, officers, nurses, academics, and private sector organisations	Developed and co-organised National Women's Health Week	Women's prison facilities	One week
Inmates	Played card games (spades), watched television, and cooked with commissary food	Multiple prison facilities (residential modules, dining halls, dayrooms)	Weekly (segment 1–5)
Inmates, education specialists, probation officers	Attended educational classes (e.g. home confinement preparation class)	Women's facilities	Two classes (segment 2)

(continued)

Table A.1 (continued)

Population/participants	Activity	Location	Duration/frequency
Inmates, officers	Observed offender intake and processing	Men's Jail and Women's Maximum	Every couple months (segment 1–5)
Inmates, nurses	Co-instructed health education classes covering sexual health, food allergies, and dietetics.	All prison facilities	Periodically as needed (segment 1–5)
Inmates, Probation and Parole Board, legal community	Observed parole hearings	Office of Parole and Probation Services	29 hearings (segment 6)

Source Author's creation

Table A.2 Prison staff participant observation

Population/participants	Activity	Location	Duration/frequency
Administrators	Observed institutional planning meetings	Administrative offices	Every couple of months (segment 1–5)
Prison Medical Director	Developed a collaborative prison-university academic course	Administrative offices	Monthly (sometimes weekly) (segment 1–post fieldwork)
Wardens, brass, and officers	Socialised in brake rooms, offices, and security substations	Multiple facilities	Weekly (segment 1–5)
Nurses	Socialised in medical dispensaries	All facilities	Daily (segment 1–5)
Administrators wardens, brass, officers, union representatives	Pharmaceutical sponsored dinners, drank alcohol, socialised outside the prison, celebrated holidays, retirement events	Melville reservation, bars, supper clubs, coffee shops, restaurants, event venues, etc	Weekly (segment 3–6)
Administrators and wardens	Informal discussions	Administrative offices	Weekly (segment 1–5)
Administrators, wardens, officers, and community consultants	Women's Prison Steering Committee	Women's facility	Monthly (segment 3–6)

Source Author's creation

Table A.3 Ex-inmates participant observation

Population/participants	Activity	Location	Duration/frequency
Ex-inmates, social workers, and outreach workers	Observed consultations between social workers, and ex-inmates, and accompanied clients to sober houses, shelters, welfare offices, hospice care, etc	AIDS Resource Centre and multiple other locations in Melville	Weekly (segment 5–6)
Ex-inmates, outreach workers	Volunteered to distribute condoms and safe injection equipment to community sex workers	Melville, West Side neighbourhood	Once (segment 5)
Ex-inmates, outreach workers	Observed home visits, accompanied ex-inmates and their social workers to community clinical appointments	Melville Hospital, AIDS Resource Centre, and multiple locations throughout Melville	Weekly (segment 5–6)

Source Author's creation

Table A.4 Community staff participant observation

Population/participants	Activity	Location	Duration/frequency
HIV consultants, ex-inmates	Observed HIV clinical appointments	Melville Hospital	Every couple of months (segment 6)
Medical physicians, medical students, and HIV service users	Observed infectious disease seminars, clinical service user groups, and medical school lectures	Melville Hospital, Melville University	Monthly (segment 5–6)
Project director, case managers, social workers, and outreach workers	AIDS Resource Centre staff meetings	AIDS Resources Centre, Melville Hospital	Weekly (segment 5–6)
Government officials, service providers, and public health specialists	Participant on a State Taskforce for HIV-prevention	Melville State government buildings	Every 3 months (segment 3–6)
Case managers, social workers, and outreach workers	Socialised at local bars, restaurants, and my home	Multiple locations throughout Melville	Weekly (segment 5–6)

Source Author's creation

Table A.5 Post-fieldwork participant involvement

Population/participants	Activity	Location	Duration/frequency
Multiple participants	I developed a semester long academic course at Melville University in collaboration with Melville prison. The course enrolled 50 undergraduate and graduate students	Melville University	Daily, 4 months (fall semester, 2013)

Source Author's creation

References

Atkinson, P., & Hammersley, M. (1994). Ethnography and participant observation In N. K. Denzin & Y. S. Lincoln (Eds.), *Handbook of Qualitative Research*. Thousand Oaks, CA: Sage Publications Limited.

Charmaz, K. (2003). Grounded theory: Objectivist and constructivist methods In N. K. Denzin & Y. S. Lincoln (Eds.), *Strategies of qulitative inquiry* (2nd ed., pp. 249–291). London, UK: Sage Publications Limited.

Charmaz, K. (2006). *Constructing grounded theory: A practical guide through qualitative analysis*. London, UK: Sage Publications Limited.

Green, J., & Thorogood, N. (2009). *Qualitative Methods for Health Research* (2nd ed.). London, UK: Sage Publications Limited.

Hong, L. K., & Duff, R. W. (2002). Modulated Participant-Observation: Managing the delemma of distance in field research. *Field Methods, 14*(2), 190-196.

Janes, R. W. (1969). A note on phases of community role of the participant observer. In G. J. McCall & J. L. Simmons (Eds.), *Issues in participant observation* (pp. 52–66). Reading, MA: Addison-Wesley.

Spradley, B. (1980). *Participant Observation* New York, NY: Holt, Rinehart & Winston.

Appendix B: Research Field

The research field comprised a range of spaces as the study followed inmates living with HIV as they moved from incarceration to the general community.

Prison

In Men's Jail, over 1,000 men resided in 16 housing modules (MOD). Each module was assigned a capital letter on the gate, and every door had "call codes" on the top right corner. Winding corridors separated the MODs across three floors. The layout of the facility was designed to easily isolate sections and minimise collective activity. Each MOD varied in size. A typical MOD had cells, a communal area, and showers. The building shared a medical dispensary, chow hall, laundry service, and intake-processing centre.

Call codes were monitored by security substations, overseen by officers who remotely controlled all facility movement. Substations were outfitted with door lock switchboards and audio and video monitoring systems.

L. Kuester, *Violence in Pursuit of Health*, Palgrave Studies in Prisons and Penology, https://doi.org/10.1007/978-3-030-61350-1

> The facility had few outward-facing windows. Fluorescent recess lighting made it difficult to determine the time of day. The space was clean, with white painted cinderblock walls, and furnishings bolted to the floor. (adapted from fieldnotes)

At the time of this research, Melville housed approximately 2,897 offenders and people awaiting trial. The institution comprised five male facilities, and two female facilities, with security levels ranging from minimum to supermax (Tables A.6 and A.7). Each facility had its own culture, movement, and staff. The fieldnote excerpt above provides an example of the physical space in Men's Jail.

The research took place in all seven facilities, as well as the Officer Training Academy, Prison Union, administrative offices, and the Probation and Parole Board. Time was spent in an assortment of spaces within each prison facility. Not all spaces were easily accessible and often depended on movement allowances in each area (e.g., free movement, segregation, protective custody). Research activities with inmates occurred in individual and shared accommodation, medical dispensary, chow hall (dining facility), prison yard, visiting centre, dayroom, chapel, barber shop, and education units.

For prison staff, research activities took place in the medical dispensary, *Med lin*e, security substations, officer breakrooms, intake-processing centres, conference rooms, and administrative offices. Additionally, I spent time with prison staff outside the Melville reservation at bars, dinners, restaurants, supper clubs, and cafes.

Filed notes depict typical interview settings in prison. For example, this was the context I interviewed Cam, an inmate in Men's Jail:

> He arrived from solitary confinement in an orange jumpsuit. He was shackled and escorted by an officer. The officer places him in a cage before I could enter the cell. Steel bars separate me from the interview participant. There is a small slot, "a trap", through which consent forms could be passes from the researcher to participant. An observation window faced toward the corridor.

Table A.6 Male prison facilities

Facility	Capacity	Average Capacity (2013)	Established	Details
Supermax	138	98	1980s	Highest security institution in the State. There were two 24-bed modules, and four 12-bed modules, and 4 hospital rooms. No industries or contact visits allowed. Most inmates reside in solitary confinement conditions. There was a medical dispensary, library, board room, barber shop, and chapel
Maximum Security	409	440	1800s	High security institution for long-term inmates and short-term inmates with behavioural challenges. There were six housing MODs, 1 segregation unit. There was a medical dispensary, dining facility, laundry, barber shop, recreation yard, education unit/gym, and industrial area
Medium Security	1006	1018	1990s	Secure "Midwest style" prison facility. There was a medical dispensary, dining facility, education rooms, and other services and other amenities
Minimum Security	710	402	1970s	Low security facility. Inmates participated in work release programmes. There was a medical dispensary, chapel, education rooms, and visitation rooms
Jail	1030	1118	1980s	High security institution for short-term inmates and persons waiting trial, or not yet sentenced. There were 16 MODs, two of which were segregation units. The facility typically processed over 15,500 inmates each year. There was a medical dispensary, dining facility, visitation rooms, and administrative area

Source Author's creation based on publicly available information for Melville prison

Table A.7 Female prison facilities

Facility	Capacity	Average capacity (2013)	Established	Details
Maximum/Medium	173	128	2000s	High security facility that housed medium and maximum-security inmates, and inmates awaiting trial (Jail). It had four MODs and a segregation unit. The facility had a dining facility, education rooms, laundry, and medical dispensary
Minimum	100	95	2000s	Low security facility. This was a dormitory style building that shared amenities with Women's Maximum. Inmates participated in work release programmes

Source Author's creation based on publicly available information for Melville Prison

Community

The research took place at AIDS Resource Centre (ARC), a case management programme for HIV-positive inmates returning to the community. I was provided with the keys to ARC and a workspace. Melville Hospital also provided a workspace and the use of a counselling room to conduct interviews with participants. The research was carried out in a range of public spaces across Melville. This included participant's homes, shelters, sober houses, hospice care community living centres, welfare offices, and State administrative buildings, as well as the public streets. While research on social workers and outreach workers was predominantly carried out at ARC, traveling to and from home visits with clients provided important time for informal conversations and observations. Bars, restaurants, supper clubs, cafés, Melville University, and the Melville Department of Health were also important research sites. Research with HIV consultants was conducted in Melville Hospital offices.

Appendix C: Participant Attributes

This study enrolled 72 participants who collectively completed 77 interviews. Effort was made to include a diverse representation of prison staff and inmates, as well ex-inmates and staff working in the community. This section provides information on participant attributes. The recruitment and sampling strategy has been reported separately.

Short—and Long-Term Inmates (n = 26)

Fifteen interviews were completed with short-term inmates (<12 months), and 11 interviews were completed with long-term inmates (>12 months).

Interviews represented 90% of all inmates living with HIV in Melville custody at the time of the study. Nine interviews were completed in Men's Jail; 5 in Men's Medium; 4 in Men's Minimum; 3 in Men's Maximum; 3 in Women's Maximum; 1 in Men's Supermax, and 1 interview with a Federal inmate in Men's Jail.

L. Kuester, *Violence in Pursuit of Health*, Palgrave Studies in Prisons and Penology, https://doi.org/10.1007/978-3-030-61350-1

The average age of participants was 40 years old (25–56). Twenty-three participants were male, and three were female. Based on self-reported race and ethnicity, 9 identified as Black, 9 Caucasian or white, 4 Hispanic/Latino, and 4 Other. The offences described by inmates as leading to their current incarceration were drug-related crimes (n = 11), violent crimes (n = 7), non-violent or not specified (n = 5), and parole violation (n = 3).

Frontline Prison Staff (n = 23)

Interviews with staff were conducted across all prison facilities. This including security (officers) and healthcare personnel working day and night shifts. Senior as well as trainee staff were represented. Healthcare staff comprised 11 nurses; 1 nurse practitioner; 1 psychiatrist, and 1 public health specialist. Eight healthcare staff were female, and 6 were male. Five staff worked in Men's Jail; 2 in Women's facilities; 2 in two-to-three prison facilities; 1 in Men's Supermax, and 1 in all prison facilities. Security staff (n = 9) comprised 4 correctional officers; 2 wardens; 2 deputy wardens, and 1 captain. Five security staff were female, and 4 were male. Four staff worked in Women's facilities; 2 in Men's Jail; 2 in Men's Maximum, and 1 worked across multiple prison facilities.

Prison Administrators (n = 8)

Administrators included: 1 senior representative of the officer training academy; 1 union representative and former correctional officer; 1 medical programmes director; 1 director of rehabilitative services; 1 director of nursing; 1 director of healthcare services; 1 chair of the probation and parole board, and 1 director of Melville prison.

Ex-Inmates and Community Follow-Up (n = 14):

Eight interviews were completed with HIV-positive ex-inmates living in the community (>12 months). All participants were previously enrolled at the AIDS Resource Centre, 6 were with men and 2 with women. Six interviews were completed as follow-up interviews with short-term inmates recruited in prison. All these follow-up interviews were with men; 3 released from Men's Minimum, 2 released from Men's Medium, and 1 from Men's Jail. Two of these participants brought a partner to the follow-up interview, which included 1 male partner and 1 female partner.

Community Staff (n = 6):

Six interviews were completed with community-based staff. Participants included: 2 social workers and 1 outreach worker; 1 outreach specialty nurse, and 2 HIV medical consultants.

Appendix D: Sampling and Recruitment

The sampling and recruitment strategy varied by the study population. Purposive sampling was used to select a range of institutions, people and spaces that represented the experience of HIV-positive individuals before, during and after incarceration. Theoretical and opportunistic sampling techniques were used to recruit prison staff and administrators from a range of facilities. In the community, purposive sampling was used to capture both staff and ex-inmates.

HIV-positive inmates were identified during twice-weekly HIV clinic that took place in all prison facilities. Prior to each clinic, I met with a public health nurse who determined the rota for inmate consultations on a given day, and which facility ran clinics. The HIV medical consultants introduced me to HIV-positive inmates and ask if they would like to participate in research. No one declined to participate.

Interview recruitment of inmates living with HIV was done through HIV medical consultants. Two inmates initially declined to participate in an interview, one of which agreed to participate during a subsequent sentence. Another inmate agreed to participate in an interview but was

L. Kuester, *Violence in Pursuit of Health*, Palgrave Studies in Prisons and Penology, https://doi.org/10.1007/978-3-030-61350-1

released before the interview could be completed. Instead, this participant enrolled as a community-based participant. A third participant did not speak proficient English and was excluded. All short-term inmates, those with less than 12 months remaining on a sentence, where offered follow-up interviews 4–8 months after their inmate's release from prison. These participants were also given an opportunity to bring a family member, partner, or caregiver to the interview. An effort was made to include a diverse representation based on length of sentence, gender, and prison classification.

Staff where sampled through ethnographic immersion, as well as for their specific role in the institution. In some facilities, staff were recruited during morning "roll call", a designated time when the study was introduced to participants. An effort was made to include staff from different work shifts, new and experienced staff, and staff doing a range of different jobs in the prison.

HIV-positive ex-inmates living in the community for one year or longer were recruited through case managers at the AIDS Resource Centre (ARC). This was done using a caseload roster. Effort was made to include a diverse sample based on length of time in the community, gender, and past classification in the prison system. Case managers invited potential to participate in the study. Theoretical sampling was done to include all staff affiliated with the AIDS Resource Centre and the HIV medical consultants to Melville prison.

Appendix E: Empirical Data and Analysis

This study produced three types of data, including interview transcripts, fieldnotes, and material documents. "Self-reflection" interviews were carried out during data collection. Tables A.6 and A.7 provides a summary of the data. All data were collected and analysed by a single researcher and regularly reviewed by a research advisory committee. Data were digitised and stored in accordance with ethical standards, which included delinking personal identifiable information from data and storing it on a password-protected computer. Paper consent forms and linked information sheets were stored in a locked filing cabinet within the university (Tables A.8 and A.9).

Data Analysis

Throughout fieldwork, data analysis "fracture points" guided who was included in the study and what questions were asked of participants. This involved preliminary coding of data and the review of fieldwork

L. Kuester, *Violence in Pursuit of Health*, Palgrave Studies in Prisons and Penology, https://doi.org/10.1007/978-3-030-61350-1

Table A.8 Interview transcripts

Interview classification	Number of transcripts (N=77)
Short and long-term inmates	26
Prison healthcare staff	14
Prison security staff	9
Prison administrators	8
Follow-up interviews with inmates in the community and ex-inmates	14
Community healthcare and social work staff	6

Source Author's creation

Table A.9 Fieldnotes & material documents

Source	Pages, documents, and audio files
Handwritten field notes	285 pages
Material documents (e.g. procedural documents, letters, meeting memos, institutional regulations)	93 pages
Artwork, poems, and letters	38 documents
Self-reflection interviews	10 audio files

journals in order to inform data collection. Preliminary coding of interviews involved a rapid review of audio recordings to identify emerging themes. Hand-written journals documented HIV clinical observations, informal conversations, daily routines, relationships, descriptions of physical space, language, and institutional rules. "Self-reflection" interviews also established emerging themes and documented my evolving understanding of the research space.

All interview transcripts, along with digitised field notes, were uploaded onto NVivo 9 software before data analysis commenced. The first step in grounded theory analysis is intense coding to open up potential avenues of enquiry (Green & Thorogood, 2009, p. 203). Detailed "line-by-line coding" was completed on all prison interview data. Coding was completed by a single researcher, and emerging themes were regularly checked and discussed with a research advisory committee.

Case files were created for "inmates", "prison nursing staff", "prison security staff", and "other staff" within NVivo. Data for each participant (cases) was "free-coded" under one of four files structures, from which codes were aggregated to form "tree nodes". For example, nodes for inmates captured actions (e.g. rape, child abuse, self-harm, suicide attempt). Nodes accounted for how participants assigned meaning in prison (e.g. strategic harm, agency, respect), as well as expression of emotion (e.g. anger, fear, violence, worries, deservedness). It considered participant's affiliations (e.g. gangs, race, career criminal), their day-to-day challenges (e.g. negotiating medical care), and relationships between inmates and staff. Nodes also highlighted the researcher position and assumptions during interviews.

The use of separate coding structures enabled better "content comparative methods" (Glaser & Strauss, 1967). High-level "axial nodes" were identified across the four coding structures (e.g. prison games, degradation, mattering) (Strauss, 1987; Strauss & Corbin, 1998). Axial nodes were applied across all transcripts, fieldnotes, self-reflection interview and some material documents. Other material documents were used only for context and background. Axial nodes enabled the researcher to "follow the thread" (Moran-Ellis et al., 2006; O'Cathain, Murphy, & Nicholl, 2010) and make comparisons across different data sources and participant populations. Comprehensive the "theme files" were developed around high level axial nodes. These files comprised Microsoft word documents ranging from 5000 to 10,000 words. Theme files, in turn, formed a skeleton structured for the empirical chapters of this book.

Throughout data analysis, I solicited feedback from the community of practice by discussing them with participants and presenting emerging research findings in academic forums. Additionally, a correctional officer and outreach worker reviewed drafts of empirical chapters and provided written and oral feedback, which helped build validity around the interpretations, identify any data gaps and highlight potentially disparate interpretations.

References

Glaser, B. G., & Strauss, A. L. (1967). *The discovery of grounded theory: Strategies for qualitative research.* Piscataway, NJ: Albine Transaction.

Green, J., & Thorogood, N. (2009). *Qualitative methods for health research* (2 ed.). London, UK: Sage Publications Limited.

Moran-Ellis, J., Alexander, V. D., Cronin, A., Dickinson, M., Fielding, J., Sleney, J., & Thomas, H. (2006). Triangulation and integration: Processes, claims and implications. *Qualitative Research, 6*(1), 45–59.

O'Cathain, A., Murphy, E., & Nicholl, J. (2010). Three techniques for integrating data in mixed methods studies. *British Medical Journal, Research Methods & Reporting, 341*, 1147–1150.

Strauss, A. L. (1987). *Qualitative analysis for social scientists.* New York, NY: Cambridge University Press.

Strauss, A. L., & Corbin, J. (1998). *Basics of qualitative research: Grounded theory procedures and techniques* (2nd ed.). Thousand Oaks, CA: Sage Publications Limited.

Appendix F: Welfare and Medical Benefits

See Table A.10

L. Kuester, *Violence in Pursuit of Health*, Palgrave Studies in Prisons and Penology, https://doi.org/10.1007/978-3-030-61350-1

Table A.10 Welfare & medical benefits

Programme name	Overview	Basic eligibility requirements for application	Medical coverage	Monetary support (amount in USD)	Duration/renewal of benefits
General Public Assistance (GPA)	State-funded programme that provides basic cash assistance and limited medical coverage to those who qualify.	• Must be between 19 and 64 years of age • Must qualify as disabled (have a diagnosed illness, injury, or medical condition expected to last 30 days or more) • Must be unable to work • Must be a U.S. citizen or legal immigrant • Must have a monthly income of $327 or less (Supplemental Nutrition Assistance Program (SNAP) excluded) • Must demonstrate financial resources (total bank assets) of less than $400), and may have only one automobile valued at less than $4,650	Generic prescription drugs only	Recipients are eligible to apply for a hardship fund worth up to $200 every three months. This money is not guaranteed automatically, and an applicant will need to reapply (through a paper application) every three months during the enrolment period	• Medical benefits will last for six months and may be renewed for another six months. • After one-year recipient must reapply for all benefits, • Benefits are revoked if a recipient is incarcerated

Programme name	Overview	Basic eligibility requirements for application	Medical coverage	Monetary support (amount in USD)	Duration/renewal of benefits
		• Adults pregnant or with children (dependents under the age of 18) are not eligible			
Medical Assistance (MA)	A state and federally funded programme known as "Medicaid". This package will cover doctor visits, medication, and hospital stays	• Must be 21 years of age or older • Must be ineligible for Medicare, Children's Health Insurance Program (CHIP), or other health insurance provisions	Doctor visits, medication, and hospital stays	Some recipients are eligible to receive monetary supplements from the [name redacted] Fund, which provides $200 per month	• Medicaid reviews eligibility status annually. During the review process a recipient may need to provide new documentation for income and assets. Medicaid determines a recipient is no longer eligible for support. The recipient will receive a letter that explains the reason for the denial. The decision can be appealed but requires a judicial proceeding with additional legal costs

(continued)

Table A.10 (continued)

Programme name	Overview	Basic eligibility requirements for application	Medical coverage	Monetary support (amount in USD)	Duration/renewal of benefits
		• Must be a U.S. citizen or legal immigrant • Must demonstrate medical need (e.g. pregnant, or a caretaker of a dependent child under age 19, blind, disabled, or have a family member in the household with a disability) • Must demonstrate that financial resources (total bank assets) are below $4000 per single individual in a household • Must have an SSI application pending			• Benefits are revoked or suspended if the recipient is incarcerated

Programme name	Overview	Basic eligibility requirements for application	Medical coverage	Monetary support (amount in USD)	Duration/renewal of benefits
Social Security Disability Income (SSDI)	A state-funded welfare programme that offers monthly payments based on disability (funds are determined by the recipient's work history). Medical coverage is provided through Medicaid.	• Must demonstrate the first three points in the Medicaid eligibility criteria (listed above) • Must demonstrate a 10-year working history • Must have little or no income and few resources (this means that the value of things owned must be less than $2,000 for a single person, or less than $3,000 for a married person)	Doctor visits, medication, and hospital stays	• A weekly wage based on an injured/disabled worker's average earnings before the date of their disability • The compensation rate is equal to 75% of their spendable base wage (in other words, 75% of a recipient's net take-home pay) • Persons with a full disability status will receive an additional $15 per week	• Total disability is indefinite compensation. Partial disability is set to expire within 6 years of the start date, at which time a recipient will need to demonstrate a continued need for disability benefits • Benefits are revoked or suspended if a recipient is incarcerated

(continued)

Table A.10 (continued)

Programme name	Overview	Basic eligibility requirements for application	Medical coverage	Monetary support (amount in USD)	Duration/renewal of benefits
Supplementary Security Income (SSI)	State-funded welfare programme that offers monthly payments for disabled persons regardless of their employment history. Medical coverage is provided through Medicaid	• Must demonstrate the first three points in the Medicaid eligibility criteria (listed above) • Must demonstrate little or no income and few resources (this means that the value of things owned must be less than $2,000 for a single person or less than $3,000 for a married person)	Doctor visits, medication, and hospital stays	A single person will receive a monthly financial stipend of $710.00 (Note: this amount decreased from $714.00 in the fiscal year 2012)	• A recipient is subject to periodic reviews to establish that they still meet the programme's income and resource limits • All benefits are revoked or suspended if the recipient is incarcerated
AIDS Drugs Assistance Programs (ADAP)	Federal government support specifically for purchasing HIV-related medication	• Must be HIV-positive • Must be a resident of [Melville] (immigration status does not matter for this program)	HIV-related medications only	No financial assistance	• This programme requires a renewal application every 6 months • Benefits are revoked or suspended if the recipient is incarcerated

Source Author's creation based on information provided by the AIDS Resource Centre. This table depicts common welfare benefits in Melville from 2011–2012

Author Index

L. Kuester, *Violence in Pursuit of Health*, Palgrave Studies in Prisons and Penology, https://doi.org/10.1007/978-3-030-61350-1

Index

L. Kuester, *Violence in Pursuit of Health*, Palgrave Studies in Prisons and Penology, https://doi.org/10.1007/978-3-030-61350-1

The manufacturer's authorised representative in the EU is Springer Nature Customer Service Centre GmbH, Europaplatz 3, 69115 Heidelberg, Germany. If you have any concerns regarding our products, please contact ProductSafety@springernature.com

Printed and bound by CPI Group (UK) Ltd, Croydon, CR0 4YY
30/09/2026
02225698-0002